PRAISE FOR
I WILL LOVE YOU FOREVER

The raw, vulnerable, and profound stories Cori shares in *I Will Love You Forever* reveal the true heart of a woman who earnestly believes God uses ordinary, flawed people for His extraordinary, perfect purpose. Cori beautifully portrays how she and her family have found that in giving yourself away to love God and others first, you just might find a purpose big enough for your life. If that is the desire of your heart, *I Will Love You Forever* is a must-read.

–Jeff Jaeger, Senior Pastor at
Crossroads Community Church

When I first asked Cori Salchert how she handles the pain that accompanies the love she pours into dying babies, she told me her heart was like stained glass—cracked and splintered from having loved and lost, but all the more beautiful thanks to the joy of having had these little ones in her life. In *I Will Love You Forever,* Cori boldly shines light through the broken places in her family's story and creates a stunning work of art that truly reflects the tears, love, hope, and heartbreak she, her husband, and her biological children have experienced while welcoming dying children into their home. *I Will Love You Forever* is a must-read for anyone who could use reminding that there is abounding beauty left in the world.

–Terri Peters, Contributing Editor at TODAY.com

Ronald McDonald House Charities of Eastern WI, provides a supportive and comforting place to stay for families like Cori's. Her tremendous story captures the variety of emotions—pain, fear, joy, and peace—that families experience when going through a difficult medical journey with their child.

–Ann Petrie, President/CEO of Ronald McDonald House Charities® Eastern Wisconsin

I Will Love You Forever is a tremendous testimony to how we can find deep meaning and purpose in suffering through the glory of God. Cori's family wrapped around my heart, and her words of struggle and redemption were a gift to read. Through Cori's powerful stories, we learn how periods of waiting in our lives give us the courage to steadily trust the way God moves and works. In *I Will Love Your Forever,* Jesus' light shines through the broken places, leaving you hopeful and encouraged!

–Courtney Westlake, author of *A Different Beautiful*

I WILL
LOVE YOU
FOREVER

Dear Bill,
   What a ride it's been!
Yes, I can be a total
psychotic but you roll
with my crazy &
honestly only God
could've known it
would have global
appeal. Thank you ♥

Emmalynn, Charlie & T.Bear

I WILL LOVE YOU FOREVER

A True Story about Finding Life, Hope & Healing

*While Caring for **Hospice Babies***

CORI SALCHERT

WITH MARIANNE HERING

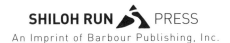

SHILOH RUN PRESS

An Imprint of Barbour Publishing, Inc.

Scripture quotations marked NLT are taken from the *Holy Bible*. New Living Translation copy-
right© 1996, 2004, 2015 by Tyndale House Foundation. Used by permission of Tyndale House
Publishers, Inc. Carol Stream, Illinois 60188. All rights reserved.

Scripture quotations marked AT are the author's translation or paraphrase.

Scripture quotations marked ESV are from The Holy Bible, English Standard Version®, copyright
© 2001 by Crossway Bibles, a publishing ministry of Good News Publishers. Used by permission.
All rights reserved.

Scripture quotations marked KJV are taken from the King James Version of the Bible.

Scripture quotations marked MSG are from *THE MESSAGE*. Copyright © by Eugene H. Peterson
1993, 1994, 1995, 1996, 2000, 2001, 2002. Used by permission of NavPress Publishing Group.

Scripture quotations marked NASB are taken from the New American Standard Bible, © 1960, 1962,
1963, 1968, 1971, 1972, 1973, 1975, 1977, 1995 by The Lockman Foundation. Used by permission.

Scripture quotations marked NIV are taken from the HOLY BIBLE, NEW INTERNATIONAL VERSION®.
NIV®. Copyright © 1973, 1978, 1984, 2011 by Biblica, Inc.™ Used by permission. All rights
reserved worldwide.

Scripture quotations marked NKJV are taken from the New King James Version®. Copyright ©
1982 by Thomas Nelson, Inc. Used by permission. All rights reserved.

Cover design: Greg Jackson, Thinkpen Design
Cover photograph: © Annabel Clark

Published by Shiloh Run Press, an imprint of Barbour Publishing, Inc., 1810 Barbour Drive,
Uhrichsville, Ohio 44683, www.shilohrunpress.com

Our mission is to inspire the world with the life-changing message of the Bible.

 Member of the
Evangelical Christian
Publishers Association

Printed in the United States of America.

DEDICATION

To Sister Jamesine, cousin Polly, and friends Liz, Mary, Ivona, Shirley, Beth, Marlene, and Faith, who have told me for years that I should write a book. I finally did.

To Bonnie and Rod, and their Sunday school of sweet little prayer warriors at Gospel Tabernacle Baptist Church: Your support over the years is precious to me.

To the pastoral staff at Crossroads Community Church in Sheboygan: Your vision and encouragement to reach those around us in our sphere of influence with the Good News of Jesus Christ is priceless and exactly what was needed to give direction and flight to our particular dream of caring for these kiddos!

To Jessica, Jack, and Bill: You've rolled with my kind of crazy and accepted the support role required with grace, and a huge scoop of humor.

To Kia and Rosie, who love my Charlie and have gone above and beyond the call of duty.

To Dr. John Piper: You didn't record all those messages about suffering and the sovereignty of God with me in mind, but God knew I needed them, oh yes, He did.

To Beth Moore: Your Bible study on Esther has forever changed my way of dealing with fear. "If this. . . Then God, then God, then God!" Thank you!

To Pete, Sarah, Bev, and Paul: Your gift of the means to go to Sanoviv the first time has had exponential results.

To Drs. Francisco, Armonia, Fernando, John and Dawn: That you find my health challenges fascinating and not frustrating is such a relief!

To Caitlin, Charlie's first foster mom: Your unshakeable belief in Charlie's value, declaring to everyone who met him, "Isn't he amazing?!" and all those prayers believing God was going to show the world Christ's love through this baby who is unable to speak, just wow! You loved our buddy first, and we're so thankful for your influence in his life!

To Jay, Steve, Keith, Kelly, John, Paul, Anne, Gordy, and all the others involved in creating a beautiful Hospice Room in our home. Our gratitude knows no bounds!

To my parents, for giving me life.

ACKNOWLEDGMENTS

Thank you. . .

To Leah from the Sheboygan Press: I am so thankful we were introduced.

To Terri from TODAY.com: You stepped back to let me tell my story. Your humility is a gift!

To Tiare from *People* magazine, who fought to convince me our story should be shared with the world.

To Jennifer Chen Tran, who believed there was a story worth telling and tangibly stood her ground in spite of the waves of doubt and fear I expressed about having anything worthwhile to say.

To Gordon Warnock from FUSE Literary, who took the risk to make the call and start this journey.

To Kelly at Barbour, who has been an encouragement and a steady cheerleader.

To Marianne, who took my pedantic drivel, which might have been solid but lacked the magic a publisher wanted. If there is anything amazing or great about this book, it's because of your influence. I've not only gained a co-writer, I've gotten a friend, and a sister in the bargain.

CONTENTS

1

BEAUTY IN THE BROKEN

O Lord, my best desire fulfil,
And help me to resign
Life, health, and comfort to Thy will,
And make Thy pleasure mine.

—William Cowper, "Olney Hymns"

The first time I laid eyes on the unnamed baby girl, I fell in love.

It was on a Tuesday in August, and the infant was swaddled in a pastel blanket and lying in a standard-issue wooden hospital crib on wheels. She was so still I found myself gazing intently at her chest to see if she was even breathing. She was not making any sound. No crying, no cooing. Her eyes were closed, and she was seemingly unaware of the medical staff bustling about, attending to the other infants requiring immediate attention in the neonatal intensive care unit (NICU).

I had been told over the phone that this tiny two-week-old girl was expected to die at any moment, and I guessed that was the reason there was no flurry of activity or staff hovering closely over her. She was not a typical NICU patient from the looks of her or the traditional crib in which she rested. The other babies, lying in isolettes or radiant warmers, were surrounded by equipment that flashed and beeped. These at-risk infants had wires and tubes attached all over their tiny bodies, and the nurses were expending great effort to make sure they would survive. The lack of life-support apparatus surrounding this particular baby was a telltale sign she was ready to be moved out of this high-energy, high-tech environment. And I was there to move her.

I exercised a great deal of self-control by reining in my eagerness to hold her by waiting about three seconds before I asked for permission to pick up Emmalynn, the name we decided to give her. The nurse assigned to her for the p.m. shift agreed with a cheerful nod that I could. I leaned over the crib, my breath catching in my lungs, a sob in my throat, tears pricking my eyes. I thought, *Oh God, is this really going to happen?* Then I carefully scooped Emmalynn into my arms and snuggled her close.

I took a breath, catching a whiff of the sweet, distinct newborn scent mingled with Johnson's baby shampoo. Baby Emmalynn was almost feather-light, and her fragility added to my desire to gather her in close and protect her.

Holding her near me and peeking underneath the typical nursery blue-and-pink striped cap, I could tell that her head, although abnormally tiny, was formed with an intact skull and a downy covering of light brown hair. My eighteen-year-old daughter, Johanna, had driven the eighty miles with me to the hospital. This was our initial visit, and I wasn't exactly sure what the protocol was or what Johanna and I would be expected to do. The nurse brought us some guest chairs, and we sat so we could dote on the precious infant. I gently ran the back of my first finger across her smooth pink cheeks.

A neonatologist wearing the usual wrinkled and faded blue scrubs came into the nursery and pulled up a stool next to us. She leaned against the edge of Emmalynn's crib and cocked her head to the side, brows furrowed in concentration and caution. "How did you get into this situation?" she asked.

I think it was a little hard for her to believe we had willingly volunteered to care for this baby. Or perhaps she thought we hadn't understood the gravity of Emmalynn's prognosis. I quickly explained that I had experience as a neonatal nurse as well as a bereavement specialist offering hospice care to families when their babies died on the labor and delivery floor. I shared my desire to come alongside an infant with Baby Emmalynn's lethal condition. I couldn't change the fact the baby would die, but I could care for her and love her for the short time she had on earth.

Once the physician realized I wasn't going to be deterred from taking the baby home, she sat back, relaxed her shoulders in relief, and grew tearful. She said, "When this baby arrived in the NICU two weeks ago, I was so dismayed because I thought she would never have a family. I'm so relieved this is happening. I don't know if you're a person of faith, but you're a godsend for this baby." She had other infants to attend to, so she left us to bond with the newest addition to our family.

Though I didn't want to hand her over, I needed to share, so I cheerfully placed the precious bundle in Johanna's arms. She was beautiful to us, and so still, like a porcelain doll. Johanna held her as gently and carefully as she could while I plied the nurse with more questions about Emmalynn's care routine. I wanted to know everything. I had already decided to give her my all, no holding back, no regrets. This baby was not going to feel the least bit unwanted. For whatever time she spent in this world, my family would give her open arms and open hearts. God had numbered her days before the beginning of time. He was fully aware of when she would be called home. I was confident He would carry us through whatever lay ahead.

After holding the precious infant one last time that evening, I gently placed her back in the wooden crib, promising that, God willing, we would be back soon. We left the NICU hoping and praying this baby would live long enough to come home.

Earlier on the same sunny day, I had been required to empty my hands of a job I had held dear. After a year of being unable to work because of health issues, I returned to the office of my former employer, a hospital on the eastern coast of Wisconsin, and met with HR staff to collect the personal items I had left behind the previous summer—boxes of photos, mugs, books, and mementos such as a hand-crocheted angel and a plaster-of-paris cast of a baby's foot. I was no longer a confident employee walking through the halls with purpose; instead, I felt beaten down and discarded.

I did not want to keep the appointment; the internal resistance I felt over this door closing in my life was stifling. Fortunately, I didn't have to go into the hospital by myself. My husband, Mark, drove me to the employee parking lot and came inside with me, expressing one of his trademark sentiments as we walked: "I cannot carry it for you, but I can carry you." His presence was steadying, and I said a silent prayer thanking God for Mark's loving support.

Stepping through the automatic doors, I realized the

grief was as fresh as it had been ten months before when I learned that the funding for my job had been redirected. There would be no job for me to come back to even if I ever did become well enough to work.

We passed by the office that had once been mine; it was now being used by a different department. Files that I had deemed of utmost importance now languished in boxes stacked on the desk in my old cubicle until someone could find the time to move them to more permanent storage.

My job as a bereavement specialist had been one of my passions. I had even come up with the program's name: Hope After Loss Organization (HALO). I had spent countless hours and had poured a significant amount of personal energy into championing the rights of miscarried and stillborn babies, and those infants who died shortly after birth, as well as their parents. One of my goals was to see that those little ones were treated with dignity and respect.

When the OB doctor needed to tell a mother her baby no longer had a heartbeat or was going to be imminently delivered and wouldn't survive, I was called. If it was possible, I would be present when the doctor shared this news, and I stayed with the family after the physician left to tell them what next steps they needed to take.

My job entailed helping parents make the best choices for their family. While the parents were dealing with the grief of their baby's death or impending death, I informed them of their options. Making funeral arrangements is horrible to contemplate, especially only hours after you thought you were going to take home a normal, healthy child.

One remarkable afternoon a baby boy was born alive after only eighteen weeks' gestation. His parents were completely overwhelmed by his untimely birth and seemed to be in shock during the delivery process. After the baby boy was born, the doctor placed him on a blue sterile cloth and handed him to me, his arms and legs gently wiggling. I had no clue how this was physiologically possible given the immaturity of the baby boy's lungs.

Seeing their tiny son moving but knowing he would die quickly was too much for the parents to bear. The boy's mother sobbed, choking out words between ragged breaths. "Please, take him away. I can't do this." The father responded to the panic in his wife's voice and motioned frantically with his hands that I should move along.

I carried the baby to an unoccupied room just around the corner and stood near the window. I held him in the palm of my hand; his tiny feet were no bigger than the nail on my pinkie finger. I could see his heart beating in his chest; I could see his veins through his translucent skin. At this early age, the nerves were just below his skin, leaving him extremely vulnerable to pain because fat stores hadn't yet covered the nerve endings to insulate them. I eased onto the wide windowsill and sat, pulling my knees up toward my chest, instinctively protecting him by arcing over his precious little body, holding him in my hands only inches from my face, cradling him with the tenderest care, offering what comfort I could. The afternoon sunlight streamed in and created a serene setting. I marveled at how beautifully his tiny body was formed, and my breath was taken away by this miracle of life, in awe that one so young continued to live outside the womb.

Tears splashed on my hands even though I wasn't consciously aware I was crying. In a half whisper I sang a hymn and then "You Are My Sunshine." My voice broke when I came to the line, "Please don't take my sunshine away."

I watched as he shuddered slightly. I whispered, "Oh, baby boy, fly away to Jesus." The fluttering in his chest stopped and his color faded. When he was still, I called my friend Marie who was working downstairs and asked if she would come help me take a photo of this precious boy. I wanted his parents to have something tangible to take home with them. A photo would be a poor consolation when Mom's and Dad's arms were aching to have a baby in them, but it was something, and something in the long run might bring them comfort.

Marie came to help me with Baby Boy without flinching, even though this certainly wasn't her area of expertise. She watched as I reverently dressed him in a small handmade kimono-style robe and then wrapped him in a blanket about the size of a washcloth. The outfit and blanket had been specially created by local church women just for babies his size. The OB nurse knocked softly on the door and poked her head in, "The parents would like to hold him now. Would you take him to them?"

I did as she asked, sighing with relief that they had chosen to hold him. The parents were going to have enough heartache, and creating a memory of their son would ease some of the pain that lay ahead. After settling Baby Boy with his family, I left the room to gather my things that I had left in the empty, hallowed space near the window.

Marie was there waiting. I had reined in my emotions while I'd had to, but now my sobs broke in spite of my best efforts to control them. "I wish I could have done something for him." I groped about in my mind, sorting through options and discarding them just as quickly. "But his lungs—they were too young to work. Any medical procedure I could have attempted would have been futile. And it would have hurt him. I feel so helpless!"

Marie looked incredulous. "You're kidding me, right?" she asked. "All that baby knew outside the womb was your touch and your love. What greater gift could you have given him?"

More than anything, the parents I worked with just needed someone to feel the loss of their child as deeply as they did, a compassionate and steady presence to help them as they learned to cope with their grief.

I loved what I did and the ability to make a difference for good in such tragic circumstances. It was difficult to accept closure, to acknowledge that this job was no longer mine.

As I walked down the hall, the heaviness in my gut was awful, and it had nothing to do with the physical pain I had endured in the past year. I felt weak, drained of energy and of the wherewithal to finish the task ahead of me. On the way to the HR office, one of my former bosses greeted me, and I felt pitied. His expression confirmed, in my mind, that my prayers and the prayers of countless others that I be fully restored to health had failed. What was even more bewildering was how much of my identity was wrapped up in my bereavement counselor role, and now I felt as if my identity had been lost along with my job. One of my worst fears had been to become disabled, and now I was staring it right in the face. My heart soundlessly cried, *Dear God, how can this be Your will for me?*

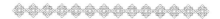

The events of the next day are proof to me that God was indeed working all things together for my good, even before I had any clue of what He was doing. Our home had passed the necessary inspection, and the initial background checks were accomplished. I had been given the go-ahead to bring Emmalynn home, and Johanna and I headed to the hospital once more, but this time we weren't just visiting. We would load this baby up in a car seat and carry our precious new gift to the rest of the family waiting at home to meet her.

On this second trip to the hospital, we found out more about Emmalynn's condition. Only the brain stem was present, which allowed her to breathe on her own, but she wasn't even able to swallow, which is a basic brain stem function. Feeding her was considered a comfort measure, and I was grateful she would not have pain from being hungry. A nasogastric (NG) tube went from her nose to her stomach so she could be fed by allowing formula to gravity feed through the tube with a syringe.

Johanna had brought with her a crocheted hat that was the color of an orange Dreamsicle from her own days as a newborn, and she fitted it over the top of the hospital-issue hat Emmalynn wore. Without this double-wrap effort, hats would fall off her tiny head.

While we were being readied for discharge, we met the neonatologist of the NICU. He was much more clinical than the physician we had chatted with the evening before. He agreed that I could use our family pediatrician, Dr. T, to provide primary care for Emmalynn. Then the doctor informed me that she was in a vegetative state. She would be almost comatose, "unable to see or hear. She will respond only to painful stimuli and have no real quality of life."

My heart rebelled at his evaluation about "quality." In spite of her extreme brain deformity and the resulting physical limitations, Emmalynn was not a mistake, as some would call her. Her body was formed in her mother's womb because God decided it would be so. I love the way the Bible describes it, saying babies are "fearfully and wonderfully made" (Psalm 139:14 NIV). God doesn't make mistakes, no matter our opinion of His work.

It honestly didn't matter one whit whether we had evidence that Emmalynn understood anything we did for her. Because she was made in the image of God, my family would be the hands and feet of Jesus and care for her as He would. This privilege of loving her even though she was too frail to reciprocate made the joy all the sweeter. God's extraordinary love for us is not contingent on our deserving it, earning it, or even, quite frankly, wanting it.

I drove home, and Johanna sat with Emmalynn in the backseat. Because she was so young and tiny, the car seat had to be rear-facing in the back, which meant I couldn't see Emmalynn's face in the rearview mirror. I was glad that Johanna could monitor the baby's breathing and alert me to pull over if she seemed to be in distress. Not that Johanna was responsible for the little baby's life—we both knew that Emmalynn could pass away in an instant—but we both agreed that if she began to struggle, it would be best for her if someone was holding her, offering comfort and love.

Having my adult daughter with me buoyed my spirits and helped to solidify that this was a team effort because I knew that on my own I wouldn't be able to provide the 24-7 care Emmalynn required. Johanna could also share in the joy of seeing a prayer honored. Three years earlier she and I had attended a Mark Shultz concert for her birthday and we heard his song "What It Means to Be Loved." Mark told the audience the song was about loving a child who most likely wouldn't live very long: "I wanna be her mom for as long as I can. . . . I wanna show her what it means to be loved." I realized that the artist had put into words what had been my heart's desire for the longest time. At that time Johanna and I had prayed for an opportunity to do just that: to be a family for a child no one else had the desire or ability to care for.

Although the dream of being able to care for babies with anomalies deemed incompatible with life outside the womb appeared to go up in smoke with the crashing of my own health, God had answered our prayers after all. We had been in survival mode for more than the past year, and my own ability to muster enthusiasm for day-to-day life was almost nonexistent. Grappling with all the loss I had experienced and feeling as if God wasn't listening to my prayers or anyone else's had taken a heavy toll. I was just going through the motions, one heavy step after another, but here, now, in this moment, Johanna could see and was reflecting a joy that I hadn't seen in her eyes in a long time.

Our prayer had been resurrected in God's timing. My husband, having once completely objected to my desire to offer palliative care in our home, was now completely on board with the plan. Our children, for the most part, were also ready and waiting to come alongside Baby Emmalynn. After a year of doubting, my heart was full of hope.

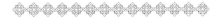

We hadn't had a newborn in the household in years. Through a couple of email messages to family and friends and some Facebook posts, word got out that we were caring for Emmalynn. To welcome the new addition, a small gathering of friends and siblings whooped and hollered when we stepped into the house. I was surprised to see a bunch of new stuff in my home. Our network's outpouring of support overwhelmed me. Friends had brought clothes and toys, and they were piled in the living room, which would double as Emmalynn's bedroom. Mary's Room, a pro-life mission organization that gives free baby supplies to their clients, also gave generously. I was looking at a just-out-of-the-box playpen covered in pink and purple flowers. We received onesies, blankets, and a gently used car seat and stroller combo.

The kids passed Emmalynn around, and everyone held her gently, some rocking her, others singing to her. I got out my phone and took photos of the event. You would have thought the president was visiting.

Andrew, my twelve-year-old, was weepy when it was his turn. "This is really sad, Mom," he said, "but we'll just hold her, right?"

"Yes," I said. "Holding her is 90 percent of what she needs."

Our eldest son, Jonathan, was very busy making a life of his own, but he came home to meet Baby Emmalynn. He normally teased and roughhoused with his sisters, but as he held our new baby girl, he showed an endearing, tender, and gentle side all of us were astonished to see.

Emily, who was almost eleven years old, remarked, "I think Jonathan loves Emmalynn as much as he loves the fridge." I agreed. Our "Refridge-a-raider"—as was his nickname—usually came to see us only when he was hungry. But he seemed to love lavishing affection on his littlest sister. After that first meeting, he was a more frequent visitor to the house and was drawn to the baby even more than he was to the contents of our kitchen.

Our girls and their friends embraced Emmalynn— literally and figuratively—without question or reserve. All of them saw themselves as her "sisters." Because of her seizures and poor breathing, we didn't expect her to sleep through the night. She would need someone close by all the time. I tried for the first few nights to have her sleep in our room. Multiple times I leaped out of bed to respond to her raspy breathing. Then I realized there was no way she could lie flat to sleep but had to be propped at a forty-five-degree angle to ease her respirations. Mark put his foot down and told our daughters they were going to help pull night duty. The girls enthusiastically arranged slumber parties so they could take on that job together, sleeping on the living room couch or floor, ready to wake me if Emmalynn needed urgent attention.

That didn't mean their work was easy. Her seizing could be unsettling and took some getting used to initially. I was proud of the way my family and our friends rallied around our fragile cherub and moved past their fears and the awkwardness of caring for a child with obvious limitations and challenges.

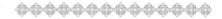

The day after we brought Emmalynn home, Dr. T stepped out of his station wagon in front of our house wearing shorts and a T-shirt. A stethoscope was draped around his neck, and he was carrying a black leather medical bag. He had cared for my kids for more than eight years, giving them umpteen well-child checkups, though we hadn't needed to visit his practice for reasons other than that. Our relationship was more based on the fact that I had known him during the years I worked at the hospital as an OB nurse. I took care of his patients when they were in the newborn nursery. We trusted each other as professionals, and we had worked well together to care for the babies at the hospital, but he had never before set foot in our home. I never dreamed he would make a house call.

When Dr. T walked inside, he seemed somber, as if he expected to find me weeping and wringing my hands over a baby in a quiet, dark, subdued setting. Instead, he found a busy, vibrant place: kids everywhere, the radio playing, a baby in bright pink clothing—and me, more animated and full of hope than I had been in months.

I lay Baby Emmalynn on a fluffy padded blanket on our dining room table, and Dr. T's mood seemed to lighten. He gave her a thorough examination. He's marvelous with kids and was gentle with the baby. She had won him over, and he seemed on board and almost happy with the plan for her care when the examination was done. He ordered oxygen because I didn't want her struggling for air, and soon after he left, the medical supply company dropped off the oxygen supplies, which included a tiny little mask with a penguin design on it, a nasal cannula to deliver oxygen via her nose should we want to do it that way, a tank for traveling, an oxygen condenser for the house, and plastic tubing.

I requested Dr. T contact our local hospice agency and have them come alongside too. He looked confused, "You know more than they do about this business. Why do you need them?"

I explained, "It's more about them maybe needing us. They probably don't have a lot of experience with a baby who is going to die at home instead of at the hospital. We can be helpful to each other."

"Okay." He complied with the request and also let the county coroner know Emmalynn was with us and to anticipate a call about her sometime in the future.

Before leaving, he gave me prescriptions for her meds: to mitigate the breathing issues and general pain, and for seizure control. Her brain stem fired erratically, and she began to rest more peacefully after the adjustments were made. Her tone was very low and her arms would lie limply alongside her body most of the time unless she was seizing.

The seizures didn't bother me, but they could alarm others. When she was seizing, her tiny hands would rise and wave about in the air. During those times, I would lighten the mood by saying, "Put your hands down, little girl, they're going to think you're Pentecostal!" which almost invariably caused the folks hearing the comment to at least smile or maybe even laugh. Our family is Baptist, though we do have moments when a little hand raising or waving during the worship service is not unusual. A sense of humor helped put everyone around her more at ease.

We were well on our way to keeping Baby Emmalynn comfortable.

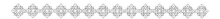

Before discharging Emmalynn, the hospital neonatologist told me she was "failure to thrive" in the hospital. He didn't necessarily think she'd live long enough to make the drive to our home. He also made me aware that should she continue to live for any length of time and gain weight, this would present a problem. Neurologically, the brain stem wouldn't be able to keep up with the demands of her growth. She was experiencing both nonepileptic seizure movement as well as epileptic seizures as the brain stem misfired.

Despite these challenges, I felt that Emmalynn was aware of me. She calmed when I talked to her and most definitely appreciated being held and touched. This was one way to calm the nonepileptic seizures. Holding her close would provide the "inhibition" necessary to stop the tremors in her body. Her eyes couldn't focus or connect with ours, but they did respond to light, so she would blink with a camera flash. She might not have had a brain present to hear or understand what we were saying, but she especially responded when Mark, her new daddy, carried her with her head tucked up under his chin so she could feel the soothing vibration of his voice while he sang to her. So we set scientific diagnoses aside and treated her like a normal human being in need of a lot of love.

We didn't bring Baby Emmalynn home to die; we brought her home to live. Because we knew her time with us would be short, my family decided to pack a whole lot of living into each day that she was alive. We hoped to make a lot of memories, and what once would have been considered ordinary activities became extraordinary because she was with us. We didn't hesitate to take our little girl to the beach, the bank, or the bookmobile.

Emmalynn's third-week birthday came and went, and she was still alive! I could tell she was gaining weight, but when she had prolonged seizures, her ability to breathe was disrupted. Even with the oxygen mask to help her recover, she would turn blue about the lips, nose, and eyes, and her lungs made a sound similar to a coffee percolator. Her struggle for air was distressing for her and for us. After a serious seizure, she would look haggard and pale, her eyes sunken. I was grateful that the medicines gave partial relief to my little girl, but they weren't completely controlling all the seizures. Mark frequently told us he hoped that she would be able to slip away peacefully when the time came.

I would nod when he voiced this request but had enough medical background to know it was highly unlikely her death would be peaceful. I thought to myself, *It's not going to happen that way, but you keep praying anyway.*

While we were conscientious about Emmalynn's health, we didn't sit around as if we were at a funeral singing dirges. Her time with us was not a deathbed vigil. In fact, since Emmalynn wasn't disturbed by loud noises as most infants are, we could play music as loudly as ever. We Salcherts do know how to have an impromptu dance party while doing dishes. We would prop Baby Emmalynn up in her bouncy chair and work away in the kitchen, singing to her or listening to the radio or CDs. She loved to be held while someone was dancing around to songs on the radio. I remember one day in particular when "I Will Survive" was playing on the radio as sixteen-year-old Charity made supper, belting out the lyrics, while Emmalynn sat in her recliner on the kitchen counter. There were certainly moments of anguish about what was coming, but the joy in each day far outweighed any gloominess over the future.

Emmalynn went everywhere with us. The older girls and I had bought tickets to see Wynonna Judd in concert. Again I followed my new rule—"Have baby, have oxygen tank, will travel"—and I dressed up Emmalynn so she could attend with us. Even without most of her brain, she did exhibit a response to sound, but she wasn't as sensitive to noise as a normal infant would be. It wasn't until the very end that she got a little antsy, and I stood in the back of the concert hall, swaying back and forth to comfort her. How gratifying it was to feel her relax against my neck and chest, cuddled in my arms.

At times I felt helpless and inept and unable to *do* much

for Emmalynn except hold her next to my heart. Was I enough? Could someone else be doing a better job of caring for her? Could someone else better anticipate her needs without feeling uncertain about whether she was having a spell, or actively dying?

I felt fiercely protective, and sometimes I would spend the afternoon in the living room with her, relieving the girls of that duty, especially when she appeared to be having the most difficult time. I would work through my fear at that point by having a conversation with myself.

"I don't think I can do this." *Well, then what?*

"If she goes to the hospital, they'll unwrap her blankets and take her clothing off to examine her. She'll be surrounded by strangers. She'll get cold, which could send her over the edge. Is that what you want?" *No, it isn't.*

"Bottom line then, what do you want?" *I want her to be in my arms when she dies, held, peaceful, and loved to the very end.*

I did not have to do this, but as a friend of mine had reminded me to stay the course, "You promised to love her through this." We were gifted with the opportunity to trust God anew, and He was going to help us do what was needed day by day.

I could not carry Emmalynn's physical disabilities for her, but I could carry her. Someone needed to be able to stay close when it was the hardest, to find the wherewithal to resist the urge to run, to stand by her even if they couldn't fix anything or change the outcome. I wanted to be brave and steady, and I prayed continually, asking for that while also thanking God we could give her the "gift of presence." She needed family to be with her more than she needed us to do things for her. I could not change the fact that she was going to die, but I was trusting that God would give me the grace and ability to mitigate her suffering when she died—and that she wouldn't be alone.

Mark called my sentimental devotion to Emmalynn the Steel Magnolia deal. I could sit and hold her for hours, and the tears might be streaming down my face because I was empathizing with her struggle for life, but if anyone had tried to take her away, saying she would be better off dying in a hospital crib, that person would have had a fight on their hands, and even if they had me by a hundred pounds, they still wouldn't have been able to take her away.

Baby Emmalynn not only brought joy to our family, she also brought spiritual comfort to those suffering grief over the death of a tiny loved one. My friend Bess and her husband, Stan, were one such couple. After years of trying unsuccessfully to get pregnant, Bess and Stan adopted children. A few months after adopting their fourth child, Bess suddenly became nauseated when she smelled smoke or bottled baby food. Sure enough, the doctor confirmed she was pregnant.

Bess loved her adoptive children, but being pregnant was a special time in her life, and she thoroughly enjoyed carrying a child and wearing maternity clothes. All went well for a few months and Bess glowed with the pride of motherhood, but then she experienced signs of an impending miscarriage. The doctor told her to stay in bed, but despite six weeks of bed rest, she went into preterm labor. Stan rushed her to the hospital where Bess was brought into a delivery room.

This was in the 1960s, and Stan was not allowed to

follow Bess into the delivery room. He was frustrated, pacing in the waiting room with the other dads despite asking several times to be able to check on his wife. Bess was given medication during delivery, which left her groggy and disoriented, but she could see a little baby in a crib just out of her reach. The nurse kept coming in to check whether the child had a heartbeat.

The nurse told Bess the child was a boy, and Bess attempted to sit up and reach toward the little baby, asking repeatedly to see Davey, which was the name she and Stan had picked out for a son. The nurse shook her head and moved the baby farther away from Bess, saying, "No, no, you'll get a picture." Bess was too weak and medicated to get out of bed on her own, and she lay back, assuming the medical staff knew what they were doing and she would at least have the picture.

The doctor and nurses never took a photograph; they didn't want Bess to have even a mental picture of her child, and they certainly didn't want her to have a physical one. Bess and Stan never saw Davey. The hospital staff decided it was not a good thing for them to be able to remember how their baby looked or felt in their arms. The staff reasoned that they would be able to forget the experience more quickly if they didn't have any memories of their dead child. Even their pastor discouraged them from having a funeral.

In recounting the events forty years later, Bess felt that everything was wrong about the way she, Stan, and Davey were treated. She and Stan never wanted Davey to slip through their lives as though he had never existed.

While I was working with HALO, Bess was free and even eager to talk with me about Davey. She showed me the white kimono with blue piping that she had carefully stitched for him but that he never wore. I gave her a beautifully handcrafted memory box as a keepsake for Davey, a redemptive offering though many years had transpired between the gift of her son's birth and receiving the gift in his memory.

Bess believed with all her heart that God had heard their heartbroken cries regarding her precious baby boy. Seeing the difference HALO made for other families experiencing the loss of a child encouraged both Bess and Stan greatly.

Soon after we brought Emmalynn home, Bess dropped a gift by the house—the kimono outfit she had created for Davey. She trusted that I understood the value of her passing this precious memento along to our baby.

One day late in September I put Emmalynn in the white-and-blue wrap. She looked adorable, so I took a few photos. Then I drove her to see Bess and Stan. It was important to me that they both meet her and have time to hold her without feeling pressured to make it quick or having anyone else vying for her attention.

As I lay Emmalynn in Bess's arms, Bess's eyes glazed with emotion—not sadness, but anticipation—as she held Emmalynn close to her, imagining how Davey might have looked wearing the precious keepsake.

Bess and Stan whispered in Emmalynn's ears, asking her to say hello to their son for them when she got to heaven. It was amazing to me how Stan, who had Alzheimer's, remembered his son who had died so many years before but during my visit repeatedly forgot who I was. He asked me a number of times, "Do you have any children?"

I told him, "Yes, I do. I have nine—eight biological

kiddos and now Baby Emmalynn."

He would nod and sweetly smile, then five minutes later he would ask me the same question again.

Bess and Stan had waited more than forty years for a memory like the one they made while holding Emmalynn that fall afternoon. I also knew they had been in the habit of praying all those years that the medical community would treat parents and babies with compassion and respect so that parents could properly grieve and heal. Tears spilled down my cheeks when I realized they had been praying for me and countless other hospice caretakers and infant advocates across the country.

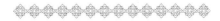

Another special piece of clothing given to Baby Emmalynn was a handcrafted knit hat. It had yellow, white, pink, green, and purple stripes; a band of purple ribbon was woven around the edge. A pretty pink flower sat as the centerpiece. The cap was too large, but I rolled up the edges and put it on over the top of the blue-and-pink striped knit hat from the hospital nursery so it would fit her tiny head.

The special gift was given to her by my friend Liz who was forty-two in August 2011. At the time she was pregnant with her eighth child, one miscarried and six live births. A 3-D ultrasound at twenty-three weeks showed the baby had no abnormalities—all measurements were perfect. She was nearly twenty-four weeks when Liz remembered having a fever, and afterward she never felt the baby move again. She believes her baby girl died during that time. Two days later she went to the doctor, and there was no fetal heartbeat.

Liz explained the gift of the hat and all the tears and prayers that accompanied it:

"I did an extreme amount of knitting after we lost our baby girl. I figured I knit over a hundred items, many for babies gone too soon. It was comforting to me, and my doctor told me it was probably because knitting mimics rocking. It was honestly what helped me through. Holding Baby Emmalynn was a huge step for me, and knowing she needed all the love that she could receive before she left this world helped me to make that step. Also knowing she would be joining my babies soon was somewhat comforting.

There was something special and innocent about Emmalynn. I knew her time was short, and as awful as it sounds now, I didn't have to envy another mom who got to keep her baby when mine couldn't stay. She helped start my journey toward healing."

For such a little squirt, Emmalynn brought much joy to my life and to the lives of others. I wouldn't trade becoming disabled for anything, because then I might not have had the honor of caring for her. Our lives were destined to intersect, and they wouldn't have if both of us had been normally and perfectly formed.

I thought of Amie, my sister whom I miss so very much. I also asked Emmalynn to carry a message to Amie—to tell her that I love her, that I always loved her, even if she couldn't understand that when she was alive. I wanted

Amie to know that I was sorry she had died alone, but I felt as though God was enabling me to make the difference now that I could not make all those years ago.

2

AMIE

I will praise my dear Redeemer, His triumphant power I'll tell,
how the victory He giveth over sin and death and hell.
Sing, oh, sing of my Redeemer, with His blood He purchased me.
On the cross He sealed my pardon, paid the debt and set me free.

—PHILIP BLISS, "MY REDEEMER"

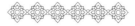

In recalling my sister Amie's life, one of the most distressing things to me is the absence of details. I have ached more at times because of what I missed in her life than what I experienced. I have heard that same ache in the voices of mothers and fathers of babies who were miscarried or stillborn. They say, "How can I love someone so much that I never met or hardly knew?" This is true for me. I hardly knew Amie, but I loved and still love her. Love doesn't end with death. One aspect of grief misses what was, and another misses what could have been. Nearly half a century has passed, and I still miss what could have been when I think about my little sister.

Perhaps the earliest memory I have of Amie was formed in Rock Springs, Wyoming. The late summer sun was streaming into our kitchen, and I sat at the Formica-topped table. My mom and dad took Amie, who was only a week old, and put her in the kitchen sink filled with warm water. But this wasn't an ordinary bath. My parents kept Amie in the warm water for a few minutes to soften the cast on her left foot and leg. Amie had been born with a clubfoot, which bent ninety degrees so that it pressed against her ankle. To gently correct the malformation, doctors put on the heavy plaster cast. After the soaking, my parents painstakingly removed the white plaster. They later took Amie to the hospital to have a new cast put on. This process had to be repeated several times during the first months of her life, and to facilitate the treatments, we moved nearer the hospital in Salt Lake City.

My next memories are snippets of Christmas Day, 1969. I was four years old. Amie was just four months old, and she was sick. Crying babies and hospital trips weren't unusual in my world. My two-year-old brother, Rob, had inner-ear troubles, which caused multiple infections. The condition also affected his balance, and he fell often, resulting in repeated visits to the ER for stitches in his head and face. I thought Amie's illness was just more of the same ol' same ol'.

No one knew just how sick she was. I have vague memories of a flurry of activity, my parents making phone calls, and the bleak darkness outside. My mom took Amie's temperature with a glass thermometer, and the mercury filled the probe to 106. That number didn't mean much to me. But my parents were worried enough to give her tepid baths and to make several calls, trying in vain to get in touch with the doctor on call. They found out later that the physician was too busy merrymaking on the holiday to answer the phone.

The next day, after reaching our family pediatrician, my mom and dad took me to the home of my mom's mom, Grandma Courtright. They dropped off Rob with my dad's dad, Grandpa Vance. Then they took Amie to the hospital.

The doctors quickly recognized symptoms of meningitis. The protective membranes covering her brain and spinal cord had become swollen and infected so badly that the doctor found it necessary to burr holes in her four-month-old baby skull to relieve the pressure on her brain. Unfortunately, no one on staff sought my parents' permission before making the holes; they didn't explain what they were going to do or why they had to do it. Perhaps it was just the way it was in 1969. They burred the holes after asking my parents to leave Amie's room and go get some lunch.

Mom came back to Amie's ICU room and found that her precious baby had a number of tufts of blood-tinged cotton sticking to the dime-sized holes in her head. When the staff explained what had been done and the reason for the procedure, Mom fainted. She was completely overcome with the suffering Amie was enduring.

Survival rates for infants with the type of bacterial meningitis my sister had contracted—meningococcal—were low. If the child survived, brain damage was almost always the outcome. During the next weeks, Amie came close to death too many times to count. Once the hospital staff gave her a blood transfusion, which she hemorrhaged right out of her rectum. After one of those near-death occasions, our family doctor sat with my mom and they cried together. He told her, "There's going to come a day when we're going to regret doing all of this life-saving of this little girl. There's nothing else that we can do."

During the three days Amie was receiving the transfusions, my great aunt Marie and a group from her California church were praying, earnestly seeking God's healing intervention on Amie's behalf. The doctors had given up hope that Amie would respond to their treatments, but she rallied, and the meningitis quit actively ravaging her body.

In February the doctors discharged Amie. The effects of the meningitis had left her brain severely damaged, causing as many as fifty seizures a day. She lost most of her hearing, her sight, and her ability to move in a coordinated fashion. Initially she wasn't able to recognize anyone. Amie was now considered *profoundly retarded*, the widely accepted term in 1970. Caring for her took much of my parents' time and attention; medical costs drained what little financial resources my parents had, and they incurred astronomical debt. There wasn't a lot of time for asking all the whys. Three children had to be taken care of, and there was no one else who was going to become chief cook and bottle washer. Simply doing the next thing required most of my folks' energy output. Dealing with the should'ves and could'ves was a useless expenditure. The question "If we don't care for Amie, then what?" had no satisfactory answer, and so they did what had to be done. Their commitments forced them to push away their anger and resentment of having a child with such great needs.

Our family valued Amie's life and deeply loved her. And that love was rewarded. Eventually Amie came to know us in a whole new way after her hospitalization. She especially "knew" my mom, in what fashion she was able to know.

My dad drove a truck, and it took him out on the road. Mom was Amie's primary caregiver, and, for the most part, the only one able to comfort and calm her. For several years my mom carried Amie everywhere, as if they were joined at the hip. Amie didn't sleep well, and consequently neither did my mom. In an effort to calm Amie and quiet her crying so the rest of us could sleep, Mom would carry Amie in her arms and walk up and down the street in front of our house. We had one sweet neighbor who would come out and walk with my mom even if it was 1:00 or 2:00 a.m. There was nothing this woman could do to relieve my sister's suffering, but she came alongside my mom and helped share in hers.

I would like to share a few memories of my folks.

We have photos of Mom wearing her hair like Priscilla Presley in a beehive hairdo circa 1965, and then a couple of years later she switched to a Marlo Thomas look from the television show *That Girl* and wore it off to the side with a flip on the ends. She had a smile so pretty she should have been a model for Colgate toothpaste. That smile covered a lot of disappointment and pain, so it was difficult for me to understand how hard her life must have been.

My dad loved music. He was self-taught on the guitar, and even after Amie's illness, he would play and teach me songs. It was a way to relieve stress, and we heartily sang "Jeremiah Was a Bullfrog" even if I wasn't totally on key.

For a long time I thought he had black hair because he used Brylcreem and slicked his hair back like James Dean or Elvis; he was every bit as good-looking as those guys. He also smoked Marlboro cigarettes. He would wear white T-shirts and roll up the cigarette pack in his shirtsleeve. He bought me packs of candy cigarettes, and I would do the same in my own shirtsleeve. We did not have seat belts when I was a four-year-old, and I rode in my dad's truck, standing slightly behind his back on the right side so I didn't interfere with his ability to shift gears. I would lay my arm around his neck and lean against him as we drove down the road. Windows down, breeze blowing through my wispy hair—Dad's didn't move, thanks to all that hair grease—we sang along to every song on the radio.

Life wasn't all sad or always chaotic.

My mom liked the house clean and orderly. Her desire was almost laughable in light of all she had to carry, literally and figuratively, but she did her best to keep the clutter at a minimum. My brother and I were allowed to get quite creative with sheets and blankets that we used to make forts.

Cooking, changing cloth diapers, washing laundry, and scrubbing dishes were never-ending chores, and my mother wore herself out attempting to keep up with it all. The money ran out long before the month was over. Amie cried almost constantly and would rhythmically and repeatedly bang her head against the floor or the crib rails or the wall. Keeping her from gnawing on her hands and arms, which left them bleeding and raw, was difficult to say the least. The stress level could be over the top, and Mom didn't have any help on a consistent basis.

At one point, social workers told my mom that they were coming to evaluate the home and our situation. Mom cleaned and straightened until 2:00 a.m. She bathed all three of us and put us in clean clothing so that everything was spick-and-span when the social workers arrived. If the social workers had found fault with the way we looked or the cleanliness of the house, the consequences could have been punitive. What an added burden!

I was too young to process all that was happening. I do remember my mom playing a Helen Reddy record album. The song "You and Me against the World" contains a poignant line: "When all the others turn their backs and walk away. . ." I now know that song probably expressed my mom's feelings of isolation as the caregiver for a child with special needs. Amie's movements were spastic, and she wailed and couldn't be consoled. Invitations to go anywhere dwindled.

Folks tire quickly under chronic duress, especially in situations that can't be fixed. It can appear as if everyone else is going on with their hunky-dory lives. My folks went without adequate rest during the night, and the energy they used up facing the relentless demands that each day brought wore them out. And there was no end in sight.

Biblical counselor David Powlison expressed the isolation that comes with caring for a disabled child: "Parents of a severely disabled child face lifelong hardships of many sorts. They also face how they are treated by others. Friends and family distance themselves or feel awkward and don't know what to say, or offer laughably (weepably?) inappropriate help, or don't want to be bothered, or offer a thousand suggestions and fixes that reveal utter incomprehension of the realities. Disability is compounded by isolation."[1]

Rob and I were too young to give my mom any support, and we could be naughty and a handful. I recall my mother telling us one evening that we had to go to bed at 7:30. I planted my feet apart, put my hands on my hips, and with all the sassiness a five-year-old can muster, declared, "I'm not tired!"

She wearily replied, "You're not, but I am. Go to bed."

Rob and I rarely went to sleep as directed; instead, we chose to romp in the bedroom we shared. Night after night my brother and I played an imagination game called "hot lava." The floor was the hot lava, and the only way to avoid "falling to our death" was to run as fast as we could across his bed, leap across the huge abyss (which was only about two feet) to the foot of my bed, run down the length of it, leap across—and round and round we'd go!

Our enthusiasm for this game got the better of us, however, because we couldn't play silently. My parents would hear our giggles and chuffing breaths, and when the beds began to creak, Dad would appear at the door.

We were not brain damaged in the same way Amie was, but we had our own brand of cause-and-effect learning disability, though it wasn't medically diagnosed. Each night we would gape at him, shock filling our wide eyes when he delivered the news that we were going to get a good-night spanking. We should have been able to figure out that our hot-lava jumping and the subsequent punishment were linked. But the next evening when it came time for bed, we would choose to repeat the previous night's performance.

I'm sure my folks scratched their heads in wonder over our inability to realize that punishment would follow our disobedience. Technically, in our minds, we hadn't gotten out of bed because we had avoided the floor at all costs!

In the fall of 1970, Mom became pregnant. During a discussion about what to name the baby, Rob suggested Superman. I thought Underdog was perfect, and my mom said, "How about Joseph Brandon?"

I wrinkled my nose, saying, "Nah! That's a dumb name." My suggestion for his title didn't count for much, and Joseph Brandon arrived on the scene in June 1971. The timing of the pregnancy seemed lousy given the craziness of my sister's health issues, but the gift of a new baby doesn't always arrive when it's deemed convenient. He wonderfully completed our family.

When Amie was three years old, her looks favored our

mother; her hair had grown in brown and curly, abundant enough to cover her scars. She had large blue eyes that were still beautiful even though at times they would roll back in her head, and the blindness made them seem vacant.

One of my favorite memories of Amie is from this era. She loved to sit on the linoleum floor in our laundry room and play with the door. There was a spring attached to the back of it, so when she swung the door toward the wall, it would bounce back to her. She was tickled at her ability to make the springy *boing* sound. Her giggle was contagious, and I laughed not because of the noise but because it delighted her so much. She would swing the door over and over and over again, never seeming to get tired of it.

Amie didn't walk on her own until she was about four and a half years old. Grandma Courtright bought her the special shoes she needed to further correct the clubfoot. Grandma also bought a wheelchair for Amie to ride in. This generous purchase helped my mom when she had to take Amie to physical, occupational, and speech therapy several times a week. The trip required at least an hour on the road depending on traffic, and Mom had three other ambulatory children to manage. Not only were we no help, but we also added stress with our disobedience.

One day my mom lost her temper with Rob and me, and she said she was leaving. Mom walked through the laundry room and went out into the garage as if to get in the car. Rob and I looked at each other, not understanding that she was trying to teach us a lesson. We were supposed to stop acting up and behave; instead, we were more delighted with the idea than we should have been.

"Let's go live with Grandpa Vance!" I suggested. "Quick,

where's the phone book so we can call him?!"

Rob found the book. I was eight then and able to read, but the way the names were arranged in the phone book confused me. I couldn't find my grandpa's name to save us. I dragged my finger up and down the columns of names, and we talked about how fun it would be to live at his house. We would eat gingersnap cookies and play in the big, old box he had in the back of his garage. It was filled with rich, black soil, and worms crawled in it by the hundreds. Grandpa sold those worms to fishermen for bait as a source of income, but to us grandkids they were just a source of entertainment. How amazing it would be to live with him!

While we were madly shuffling pages of the phone book, my mom walked back into the house and saw us. We were disappointed that she was back and that we hadn't had time to call Grandpa before she returned. Whatever lesson she was hoping to teach us about learning to behave was lost.

I'm surprised my mom didn't lose it more often. On top of Amie's health-care issues, my dad, my grandma, and I piled on ours. Dad had rheumatoid arthritis, and it was causing more pain than he could tolerate and still drive a truck. He missed more and more days of work. Grandma Courtright was prone to falling, and the resulting injuries required care. I had asthma, bronchitis, and all manner of gastrointestinal (GI) troubles.

When Amie was five years old, the American Fork Training School for the Mentally Retarded approached my parents about the idea of having Amie live at their facility. My folks were given a tour of the state-run children's home where she could live, get medical attention, and receive therapy on a regular basis. The staff of the training school would be able to help her walk, feed herself, and use the toilet unassisted. They said my sister would excel in ways that wouldn't be possible if she remained with our family.

Mom and Dad were faced with one of the toughest decisions they would ever have to make. I know my mom cried often, and both were filled with anguish. After receiving counseling from family, doctors, and friends, and praying long and hard with our church's pastor, Mom and Dad decided to put Amie into the training school. They concluded it was the best option for all involved.

At the time, I didn't fully comprehend what was happening. It seemed to me that Amie just up and disappeared. She was home one day and then gone the next. To add to my confusion, we didn't visit her. The training school had discouraged my parents from doing so, telling them not to come to the institute for months. They especially advised my mom to stay away so that Amie could bond with her new caregivers.

I'm sure my parents gave me some explanation, but I wasn't able to comprehend the myriad factors contributing to Amie's leaving. To make sense of it all, I constructed scenarios to fill in my gaps. Basically I made up a bunch of stuff that was very real in my day-to-day world. It seemed reasonable to cast the blame for our family's troubles on my shoulders. *I felt it was my fault.*

At nine years old, I certainly couldn't fathom how hard-pressed my parents were. Amie was getting heavier and more unmanageable on every front. They had to juggle the unrelenting needs Amie presented and also rear three other young children who also had health issues, care for my ailing grandma, battle my dad's rheumatoid arthritis, and deal with crushing financial burdens. I thought I was in some way responsible for my family's predicament, for whatever bad things might be happening. I have since learned that clinical psychologists call this mind-set "magical thinking." I definitely carried a load too heavy for my young heart, and I became weepy and withdrawn. I tried as hard as I could not to cry by pinching my arm or biting my lip. But the harder I worked to hold all my emotions in, the more I couldn't help myself. One of my nicknames in grade school was "crybaby." The very thing I wanted to do the least was something I seemingly had no power to stop. Most of the time, the circumstances didn't warrant the torrent of tears I could unleash, but my emotional pain was real and spilled out at the slightest trigger. If I heard it once, I heard it a thousand times from adults: "Stop crying, or I'll give you something to cry about."

I recently read Kate Larson's book *Rosemary: The Hidden Kennedy Daughter*. Rosemary was considered mentally disabled, having been injured during birth. Her father, Joe Kennedy Sr., was ill advised in his quest to get help for her. It was decided she should undergo a lobotomy to rein her in and "solve" her mental troubles. This was a disastrous solution. She left the family, and some of her siblings didn't see her for years.

The book recounts Ted Kennedy's feelings about his sister's disappearance:

> "What Rosemary's siblings were told about the surgery and its outcome has not been fully recorded, but clearly it was little. . . . Young Teddy was particularly troubled by Rosemary's sudden and unspoken disappearance from the family circle. At nine, Teddy feared that he "had better do what Dad wanted or the same thing could happen to

me." There "will be no crying in the house" Joe told Teddy and his siblings, so whatever fears Teddy harbored, he kept to himself."[2]

The enemy of my soul, Satan, used Amie's leaving to wage war in my heart for almost thirty years over my worthiness to be loved and valued. I bought his lie "hook, line, and sinker," that I had to be perfect or I would be abandoned by my family and never see them again. This was not true, and no one told me this. I figured it all out in my head and drew faulty conclusions, which I was too afraid to voice for fear they would be validated for sure if spoken aloud.

The times I was legitimately ill with breathing or intestinal issues, I was afraid my being sick wasn't okay. I compared my situation to Amie's. Her permanent brain damage and physical disabilities were real—no one ever questioned or doubted them. Anything that happened to me seemed to pale in comparison, and I felt as though my own temporary troubles were invalid because Amie's were severer. I thought my troubles weren't worth other people's concern or attention. For years I dealt with a conundrum: I needed nurturing and validation of my own hurts and fears, but I rejected myself as unworthy of receiving care and compassion when they were offered. No one but me was comparing me to Amie, but I continued doing it, consciously or not, well into adulthood.

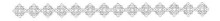

In 1975, at age thirty-one, my dad became permanently disabled. This resulted in a great deal of upheaval and several moves to find affordable housing. For us kids it meant changing schools and finding new playmates. My mom went to work, and my dad was at home with us, and because of the pain he was in, he was unable to handle a lot of noise and commotion. Basically my parents had to regroup and find another way for my dad to work. He needed a place where he could get training for a job that wasn't as physically demanding as truck driving. He requested permission from Social Security so he could attend Denver Baptist Bible College. He expected the government to turn him down flat, but the request was granted. My folks subsequently packed everyone up and moved to Broomfield, Colorado, when I was ten years old. We spent the next four and a half years there while my dad went to school and got his degree in pastoral studies.

During that time our whole family would travel back to Salt Lake to visit our grandparents and Amie at least once a year. The trip was about five hundred miles, and because the speed limit was 55 mph, the drive took at least ten hours. We usually left in the evening and drove all night. I know I'm not alone in having a strict dad who wanted to drive straight through. He did not stop driving until the gas tank had to be refilled. Now that we are adults and have children of our own, my brothers and I find it laughable that we were instructed to drink minimally because Dad was not going to pull over every half hour to let one of us kids out to pee. There were quite a few stubby pines along Route 80 in Wyoming, which received a sprinkling because the rest stops along that road were few and mighty far between.

One year my folks brought Amie and her caregiver to Colorado. My memories of this visit are fuzzy. Amie wore thick, dark-framed glasses that "corrected" her vision, but even with them, she was legally blind. When she tried to walk, she was spastic and disjointed. She cried with a loud wail that set my teeth on edge. It was especially painful because we wanted to comfort her but weren't familiar enough with her to know what was wrong or if indeed anything was wrong at all.

Our visits were infrequent and brief, but my family certainly made the effort. We didn't travel anywhere else, and with our limited income, these visits were an extravagant luxury. At times Grandma Courtright would buy me a plane ticket so I could fly back alone to visit her. She and I made it a priority to spend time with Amie at the training school whenever I was in town. Because of my own health issues, I was a skinny little thing. In contrast Amie was quite sturdy. My grandma was about as tall as she was round, and she found it a little hard to manage holding Amie's uncontrolled movements. The encounters were all a tangle of arms and legs, and Amie ended up either cackling or crying. She was a handful, and Grandma and I weren't too successful in our wrestling matches with her.

One thing that made me laugh and made my grandma frustrated was that in spite of Amie's brain damage, she knew when she didn't want to be picked up and would raise her arms above her head so there was no way to get a firm grip under her armpits. She would wriggle her way out of our grasp and be laughing herself silly while doing it.

My grandma was a stoic if there ever was one. She rarely cried, but after our visits with Amie, we would drive from American Fork back up to Salt Lake City, and there would be a moment when a tear or two would make its way down her cheek. She never failed to take me to see Amie or visit my grandfather's grave when I came to visit. Both things were hard and a source of grief to her but important enough that she continued to do what was necessary.

Whether or not it was my fault, Amie seemed disconnected from me. What I could give to her and what we could mean to each other were not enough to form a satisfying relationship. My magical thinking mind-set had not evaporated. I felt responsible for the disconnect between us. Living with regret is a heavy thing. There was no way to explain to Amie the various reasons why we didn't have much of a relationship. I didn't know her because of the lack of personal contact, and she was in no way attached to me for the same reason. I was cognizant and pained by the absence of truly knowing her, while Amie was innocent and did not carry that burden.

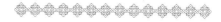

While the details surrounding Amie's life have faded, my memories surrounding her death are vivid.

In 1980 my father completed Bible college, and my folks were not altogether sure what was next. Then one of our former pastors and his wife offered to pay for our move to Sandy, Utah, where my father could help pastor the tiny congregation. So in the summer of my fourteenth year, my family left Colorado, and we moved into the church's mission house.

About a year later, on Saturday, June 6, the phone call came. I remember I was standing on the driveway. I had on shorts and a tank top. I wasn't one for wearing shoes, and so I was barefoot when the phone rang. My mom called for me to come inside, and I ran into the house, the gravel of our driveway pushing into the soles of my feet.

My mother told me and my brothers that the unthinkable

had happened: Amie had drowned.

The tragedy unfolded at a watermelon picnic on Friday evening held on the training school grounds. Amie had participated in the celebration, and a caretaker had guided her inside to use the bathroom. Since Amie was capable of doing this task herself, the caretaker left her in the bathroom alone, and then she went back out to check on the other children. Amie finished her business and left the bathroom, but apparently she did not go back out to the picnic area. Instead, she somehow found an unlocked door, which allowed her to slip out of the fenced-in property of the training school.

After she was noted missing, the police, volunteers, and the staff at the training school spent the next fourteen hours looking for her. Amie had wandered onto the adjacent golf course and drowned in a lake. I'm not sure why no one saw her. It would have been obvious from her stature and her awkward gait that she was not a golfer but a child needing supervision. Whatever the circumstances, no one intervened on her behalf.

Her accidental death had been a source of grief and anger and confusion to me for decades. Authorities don't know for sure what time she found the lake and decided to wade in. No one knows at what point she subsequently found herself unable to cope. My family has speculated that since she loved being in the pool at the training school, she most likely initially felt confident and safe splashing in the water. The terror she must have felt as the water became a death trap makes me shudder. No one has ever told me how deep the lake was near the shore. Perhaps she fell down and wasn't able to right herself. If she cried out, her voice went unheard and unanswered by human ears.

Regardless of the what-ifs, one thing is known: my little sister lost her life that day.

During the search the staff at the training school had been attempting to reach my parents by phone with no result because the number they had listed was for our home in Colorado. The social worker had our new one, but it was not on her chart at the home. We felt it was a grace given to us that they didn't have the right number. To search all night for Amie and then to have seen her lifeless body would have been horrifying. Just hearing the news she had drowned was devastating enough.

I heard the news and immediately left to go to the "back house," as we called it, which was a tiny apartment for missionaries who might be visiting our church. It doubled as a printing room. Pastor J, one of our family's nearest and dearest friends, was working back there printing bulletins for Sunday service. I was crying and trying to tell him Amie had died. He asked me to slow down, to stop blubbering a minute, and to speak more clearly. When I choked out the news in a way he could understand, he pulled me in close for a hug I desperately needed at that time.

The rest of that afternoon is a hazy memory of sad-faced family and friends reaching out to us to express their sympathies and offer comfort. The phone rang and rang, my parents relating the tragic story multiple times. In between visits and phone calls, my parents began to make funeral plans. My mother made sure my brothers and I were included in the planning process. She didn't want it to be an event where we came as spectators. My mom laid out the possibility of having an open-casket funeral. We unanimously rejected that awful idea, saying that displaying a picture on the casket would be better, leaving us to imagine her as we last saw her.

I had great fear of seeing Amie lying there not moving or making a sound. I shuddered and trembled just contemplating it, because up to that point my experience with death had been with elderly relatives.

In my estimation Amie's death was wrong on so many levels. I wasn't alone. I overheard some adults who visited tossing around words such as *negligence* and *lawsuit* and *compensation*. I don't remember my dad saying much of anything. He's not really the talker in our family anyway, but my mom fairly quickly shut down all of that mean-spirited conversation. She told our visitors that the people at American Fork Training School had cared wonderfully for my sister. Yes, the doors should have been locked, but Amie's caretaker was not at fault for her wandering off. A number of "should've's" could have been discussed, but no amount of talking would bring back Amie. Nothing could have changed the outcome, and my mom avoided expending a great deal of energy dwelling on what could have been different. I wasn't worried about placing blame, but I had a lot of unanswered questions.

I crawled into my bed with family photo albums after the initial hubbub of people had left our home. I spent hours flipping through the pages of the album, crying until I had no more tears. *Where were You, God?* I asked over and over. I felt such deep hurt over this injustice. I was scrambling in my head to make sense. *Why was she left alone? Why was the door left unlocked? Why hadn't anyone seen her? Why didn't she wander in a direction that would have been safer until she was discovered? Why? Why? Why?* The unanswered questions tortured me.

There were no answers—not viable, good, satisfactory ones, answers that could calm my soul and bring healing for the hurt. And my pain was unlike anything I had ever experienced up until that point. I knew God was able to save my sister. Why hadn't He done so? I had wanted more time with her. I wasn't old enough to drive yet, so I couldn't go see her without an outing arranged with an adult. She lived about thirty miles away, so riding my bike wouldn't cut it. I felt as though I had done so little, and now it was too late to do things differently. A heavy, crushing load of guilt descended on my weak shoulders, guilt that wasn't mine to carry as a fifteen-year-old.

My grandpa Vance came over to visit. He always wore a baseball cap and had more than a day's worth of gray stubble on his chin. He smoked like a fiend, so the smell always clung to his clothes. He would grab me about the waist, pulling me close to him, and chew on the top of my ears and give me whisker burns on my neck and cheeks. For years he told me not to swallow watermelon seeds or one would grow out of my belly button. After every evening spent on his porch eating the fruit, I would go home and check for signs of one sprouting out of my navel.

Grandpa Vance was still a favorite of mine, so his visit and words carried importance and weight with me. He sat down in a chair next to the front door in our living room, and I sat on the floor to his left so he could play with my hair, twirling it absentmindedly through his fingers. My mom was across the room on the couch. He began to talk about drowning victims, about how they were black and bloated. My mother shut him down immediately. "That's not true, Vance!" she said. The discussion ended abruptly.

I carried his comments with me for the longest time.

I wondered why he had said it if it wasn't true. I didn't find out the reality until I was a nurse with a year's work experience, sitting in a hospice orientation class at Grand View Hospital in Pennsylvania. Our instructor mentioned her husband was on a diving team that recovered drowning victims. I asked her if she knew what happened to the bodies of people who died and spent hours in water. She explained that bodies left in water become bloated and the skin can darken, even become black.

I later questioned my mother about Amie's body, and she told me Amie's social worker had no idea she was missing, and ironically, he was the golfer who came across her body in the lake. When he called to tell my mother Amie had drowned, he could hardly get the words out he was sobbing so hard. He had been able to identify Amie only by her long, curly brown hair. The rest of her body was unrecognizable. Mom explained she had shut down the discussion with Grandpa Vance to protect me. She knew I was already having nightmares about Amie. Every night I dreamed my sister was struggling and crying, with nobody coming to help her. Adding the gruesome details to my imagery would have unnecessarily added grief.

I was grateful that I found out the corporeal realities of drowning at a time when I was more emotionally and mentally capable of grappling with them. I was not any less wounded, but I was an adult. I do believe God sometimes keeps things hidden until we're in a place where they won't harm us. In holding some information back, my mom gave me a gift, and I'm grateful.

Images of Amie's death plagued me for years before I could finally assimilate that she was no longer wildly fighting for her life, wondering why there was no one to help.

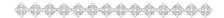

Being a pastor's child, I knew well the account of Jesus raising Lazarus from the tomb: Lazarus fell ill and died, and his family prepared his body and placed it in a cave. Days later Jesus arrived and called forth Lazarus from the tomb, grave linens and all.

I knew the basic facts of the Bible miracle, and yet I didn't fully appreciate the nuances of the account until I resonated with the grief of Lazarus's sisters. John 11 says that Mary and Martha each went to Jesus separately and said to Him, "If you had been here, my brother would not have died" (vv. 21, 32 NIV).

Those words break my heart because I understand dashed expectations. God is fully capable of stepping in and healing and preventing any illness or injury from happening in the first place. But sometimes He doesn't step in when we want Him to. The grief I read in the sisters' response is palpable. I feel the depth of their pain and disillusionment. The women were disappointed because they knew if Jesus had been there in time, He would have healed Lazarus as He had done for so many others.

Martha and Mary knew and believed Jesus cared, because their urgent message to Jesus was "The one you love is sick" (v. 3 NIV). They hoped in the fact that Jesus loved Lazarus, and they thought their brother would receive special attention from the Son of God. Surely Jesus would put effort into saving the life of His beloved friend since He had already touched the lives of countless others. Surely Lazarus's life meant more to Jesus than a stranger's. But Lazarus died despite the urgent message the women sent to Jesus. No special attention came, and Martha and Mary wailed in their despair.

But when Jesus did arrive, He wept with them.

Jesus was and is fully God, and therefore He knew the future—He knew He was going to raise Lazarus from the dead. The Bible calls Jesus a "man of sorrows, acquainted with deepest grief" (Isaiah 53:3 NLT), so He also was able to identify with Mary and Martha's pain. It's a gift to us that He is also fully human, and in the depths of His heart He can feel the pain and suffering we deal with in this life.

I have said this to God: "If you had been there, my sister would not have died."

But she did die.

In John 11 Jesus said to Martha and Mary, "I am the resurrection and the life. The one who believes in me will live, even though they die; and whoever lives by believing in me will never die" (vv. 25–26 NIV). They received their miracle within days of asking for it.

But I'm still waiting for mine. And I wait with hopeful anticipation in the promises I have today.

In 2008 I heard a beautiful song that helped me take a few more steps in the healing process. The song is "Unredeemed," performed by the group Selah, and the message is this: when something in your life is shattered, and you place it before God, He will redeem it.

For years I felt as though I could wave my sister's death in God's face and challenge His faithfulness. But just like my fears over being abandoned if I should prove too unworthy of love, I didn't necessarily voice my challenge out loud. It was a guarded area of hurt, deep and unhealed. I knew it was not acceptable to tell God I knew Him better than He knew Himself, that in some way I could find Him guilty. My perception, not unlike Job's, was skewed. Job was innocent, so he concluded that his multitude of painful trials were a result of God being unfair. God challenged this thinking in the last couple of chapters in the book of Job, and I cannot read them without the hair on my neck standing up. God is incapable of being unfair or unjust. I, like Job, will not understand everything God ordains this side of heaven, and I had best be leaving the discrepancies to Him.

I became worn out from my bitterness and wounding, and I fully believe God moved in my heart to finally ask Him to redeem the stinkin' mess. I wanted to let go of the past and stop letting it have sway over my present and my future. There is grief that pierces our souls deeply. None of the hypothetical bandages I slapped on it stuck. The healing process, if it's going to be good and lasting, cannot necessarily be sped up to meet a nanosecond tolerance for inconvenience and pain.

Finding healing has been a work in progress for me. The redemption in my life has been occurring at a snail's pace for more than thirty-five years, and it isn't done yet. But, amen and hallelujah, I can see a healthy scar forming over the festering wound that had stopped me from truly trusting God. I now know that God never fails, though it certainly seemed that He did. In a way I'm waiting for heaven, and in a way I'm living in the now. I want as much healing as is possible this side of heaven. I want to lay down all that grief or, in my case, vomit the messes in my life at the foot of the cross. I cannot even say I lay my burdens down at the foot of the cross, for the word *lay* doesn't convey the depth of the purging and healing taking place in my soul. This process gives me strength, and I cling to the knowledge that God is able to work all things together for my good (Romans 8:28). I also know that earth has no sorrow that heaven can't heal. I will not be perfectly whole and well and unwounded until heaven. When God wipes away every tear from our eyes, there will be no more unanswered "whys" from this life. I can wait until then and leave my unanswered questions in God's very capable hands.

3

FIFTY DAYS

I'm so glad I learned to trust Thee,
Precious Jesus, Savior, Friend;
And I know that Thou art with me,
Wilt be with me to the end.

—LOUISA M. R. STEAD,
"'TIS SO SWEET TO TRUST IN JESUS"

At dawn I sneaked into the living room toward Emma-lynn's infant chair, which was positioned on the floor near the couch. We had tried to have her lie flat in a crib, but it was difficult for her to breathe that way. The seat, which was covered in yellow-flowered fabric, allowed her to recline at a forty-five-degree angle. She looked like a princess sleeping on her throne.

It had been Mary Elisabeth's turn to keep nighttime vigil over her baby sister, and the fourteen-year-old was stretched out on the couch, sleeping within arm's reach of the recliner.

After having Emmalynn in our home for five weeks, I was now used to her paraphernalia being strewn about: diaper wipes, blankets, hats, and her oxygen mask with the penguin on the front. For a child who couldn't really move unless we moved her, and she only went where she was carried, having her stuff all over the house was certainly not her fault! An oxygen condenser had been wheeled into the corner of the living room, and its steady hum was almost hypnotic. Stepping past the machine, I kneeled next to Emmalynn and checked to see that the nasal cannula was positioned correctly. I noticed her mouth was dry from the added air support, so I used an oral swab to moisten her mouth. She scrunched up her face with a hilarious but endearing grimace, and I barely kept myself from laughing out loud. *So much for being a "veggie,"* I thought. *You're quite opinionated about things for not having much of a brain to work with.*

Emmalynn's color was pink and she looked fine, which filled me with relief. The day before, she had seemed off, though I couldn't put my finger on any specific reason why. I leaned over and kissed her smooth cheek, and after straightening her pink cap, I left both girls sleeping peacefully and went into the kitchen.

Mark worked second shift, which meant he didn't have to be at work until the afternoon. He was preparing his "world-famous" oatmeal for our family, which was his normal morning routine. The four school-aged kids would be up soon to eat breakfast and get their backpacks and lunches ready.

I pulled my old, comfortable hoodie over my head and slipped on my athletic shoes. I headed out the front door, jamming my cell phone into my jeans pocket. This was the only time of day I was ever gone from Emmalynn, but I still needed to be available in case something happened that Mark couldn't handle.

The air was chilly and the wind brisk. I snuggled my hands deep into the hoodie pocket to keep warm. The chill reminded me that summer was over and autumn had taken up residence, boldly decorating the region with purple, red, and yellow leaves.

As I strolled along the blue waters of Lake Michigan, the waves flirted with the shoreline, inching up the sand and then playfully pulling back. It was during these brief moments that I could think more clearly. That morning I made simple but ambitious plans to clean the house. Or maybe not. Maybe I would sit with Emmalynn and enjoy her company while the rest of the gang was gone.

When I arrived home, Mark had just finished washing the breakfast bowls. The kids gathered their school stuff together and headed out the door. A few minutes later, Johanna left to go to work. Mark went off to prepare for his day and take advantage of the few productive hours he had before leaving for work.

Suddenly I found myself with an age-old dilemma. The house needed a lot of attention since no magic fairy was going to come clean it for me, and supper should probably be prepped, too. Caring for a baby—any baby—creates a daily tension. Should you spend time nurturing the child, or should you attend to other practical duties and put the child in a safe place until your work is done?

Caring for a terminally ill baby heightens that tension, and since Emmalynn had such limited mobility, it was easy to keep her in her chair and get "important" things accomplished. Other than her fairly consistent hiccupping, she wouldn't make a peep unless her diaper needed changing.

Oh, what to do, what to do? The task list was endless, but I made my choice. I recalled a stanza from a poem that reflected what was on my heart that morning:

> Oh, cleaning and scrubbing will wait till tomorrow,
> But children grow up, as I've learned to my sorrow.

So quiet down, cobwebs. Dust, go to sleep.
I'm rocking my baby. Babies don't keep.[1]

I tossed the to-do list out of my head to focus on the baby girl right in front of me. We had places to go a little later, so for now we were going to sit on the front porch steps and soak up the sunshine warming up that side of the house. I picked Emmalynn up from her little seat and carried her outside in my arms.

The next few hours passed by at a leisurely pace. I sat with Emmalynn propped on my thighs, her head leaning against my knees, her feet resting on my belly. I felt a little desperate to memorize what it felt like to hold her—the weight of her bottom resting in my lap, the softness of her cheek. I nuzzled the skin next to her earlobe, inhaling her new-baby smell that couldn't be replicated on my own arm no matter how much Baby Magic lotion I applied.

Emmalynn had a seizure, and her little arms and hands raised in the air and waved briefly. The medications didn't stop the episodes; they only lessened the intensity. Hiccuping sessions almost always followed her seizing. I leaned back and looked down at her, marveling at her little hands, arms now lying limply at her side. Her tiny hands and fingers were curled up a bit and not entirely splayed. I took one of her hands and wrapped all her fingers around one of mine. Then I gently stroked across the dimpled area of her knuckles.

Initially I watched the traffic go by and rocked her with a gentle swaying of my legs. I sang silly songs to her like "The Wheels on the Bus" and "Old MacDonald Had a Farm." I could tell that the motion and singing soothed her.

Emmalynn was exactly seven weeks old on this Wednesday in September, but I still counted her life in days—now forty-nine—because I knew any one of them could be her last. I was thankful for each day and considered each one a near-miraculous gift given to me by God. And like Him, who counts our days and knows the number of hairs on our heads, I carefully kept track of the details surrounding Emmalynn's life and cherished them in my heart.

Before meeting Emmalynn my life had been shattered—my health and my dream job were gone. I had felt as if I had lost everything during the course of my extended illness. This wasn't entirely accurate, but God had to empty my hands or there wouldn't have been room for Emmalynn.

Three years earlier Mark had been hesitant when I had broached the subject of taking in a terminally ill child, or one with a lethal anomaly. His main objections were my full-time job, our eight children, and our numerous other commitments. He also didn't care to bring the grief accompanying a dying child, home to live with us. At that time our family didn't have enough resources to care for an infant who would require round-the-clock care. Now the timing was right.

I could not have anticipated, or wanted, the means by which my schedule was cleared so I was free to take in this sweet baby. When I had been healthy, I was busy. God knew that Emmalynn didn't need me busy. She needed me still. Accommodating my own physical weaknesses left me strong on her behalf. I could give her my presence, which was the best gift possible. She needed someone to be with her. To hold her. To love her. To be by her side when she died.

I was awed by acknowledging I wouldn't have been able to care for Emmalynn without first having endured suffering on many fronts, including the pain endured during God's silence. C. S. Lewis described the feeling as "a door slammed in your face, and a sound of bolting and double bolting on the inside. After that, silence."[2]

Until you have been there, you don't understand how crushing it is to feel you have been forsaken by God and been left in "a terrifying darkness" like the patriarch Abraham (Genesis 15:12 NLT).

When it was so black, I wondered why God just seemed to up and disappear, leaving me alone. Once upon a time I would have attempted to argue with someone who thought God had removed His comforting presence, but not anymore. I thought I could bear anything as long as I still had the sense of God's presence, but He took even that away.

I sat on my porch holding Emmalynn and wept. I was no longer shattered, but I still ached with how intensely difficult the pain had been. I know Christ was never so alone as when He was on the cross, and yet He couldn't have been any more in the center of God's will than He was in that moment.

Knowing that my Savior had been touched with the grief and sorrow I had experienced was comforting, even though I didn't have answers for why it had all been so intensely difficult.

My phone dinged. I received a text that made me grateful that Emmalynn's life had had such a beautiful impact on so many others. A widower had recently stopped by to hold her. He had sent a message thanking our family for letting him visit. He had grieved more deeply on the one-year anniversary of his wife's death than he had expected to and said holding our baby girl was healing for him. He had texted: "To my friend, Emmalynn, you're a wonderful reminder to anticipate the future and to look toward heaven."

The time on the porch had flown by quicker than I could have imagined, and we had places to go. I changed Emmalynn's diaper and her clothes, choosing a pink, hooded coverall that had belonged to Emily, my youngest daughter. In the short time we'd had her, Emmalynn had become one of us.

Before we could go anywhere, she needed to be fed. She had come to us weighing just about six pounds. She had gained two pounds-plus in a month. We weren't overfeeding her, but because of her inactivity, she soon filled out. Using a large syringe without the plunger, I introduced some formula into her NG tube, and gravity allowed the food to reach her stomach. Her body accepted the nourishment.

I knew that every ounce of weight she gained placed a strain on her brainstem, and the irony was not lost on me. Emmalynn would not be able to keep up with the neurological demands her growing body would make.

After lunch was done, I gathered everything together to make our trip. I shoved ordinary stuff like baby wipes into her diaper bag, but I also included her medications, syringes, and additional feeding tube supplies. I threw the bag over my shoulder along with my purse, which contained everything but the kitchen sink. With my left hand I rolled the frame of the large green oxygen tank behind me, the long tubing coiled around the handle. With my right, I carried Emmalynn, who was nestled into her car seat. We were armed for bear to say the least!

I had an appointment with an occupational therapist in a last-ditch effort to improve some of my health challenges.

The medical office was seventy miles away, and hiring a babysitter was not an option. I always took Emmalynn with me. Because of her fragile health, I was unwilling to be far from her side. My motto had been amended to include Emmalynn's accouterments, "Have baby—and oxygen tank—will travel."

The trip was not long unless you were a baby who couldn't move to get the pressure off her bum. Sitting in her car seat for an hour to get to the hospital probably was uncomfortable for her, but she didn't get fussy. She never did. If her diaper was full, she might whimper like a kitten mewing, but that was the extent of her demands.

Acquaintances either oohed and aahed over Emmalynn or pulled back and away, their faces registering discomfort. The therapy staff at the medical facility knew she had a lethal condition, and they understood the need to bring her along to my appointments. Some appeared to be compassionate toward her and the role my family was playing in her life. Others probably thought I was a little nuts. I noticed some staff members ducking into empty rooms in the hallway, possibly to avoid contact with Emmalynn and her tubes and conspicuous oxygen tank.

Emmalynn was unusually quiet and motionless during my therapy session, and it made me feel wary. It was the second day in a row she had been off. Yesterday a friend had remarked that my countenance seemed sad, and today my heart was just as heavy.

I nuzzled her cheek and whispered, "What are you doing, sweetheart? This is uncharted territory for me."

After the appointment I loaded the oxygen tank, bags, and Emmalynn into the car. I stood for a moment paralyzed by indecision. I was in a quandary I had never encountered in caring for a baby. The baby's car seat had to remain in the backseat according to child-safety guidelines. And it had to be facing the rear of the car, so I couldn't monitor her using the rearview mirror. A friend had promised she was getting one of the infant mirrors you can hang over a rear headrest, but she wasn't going to bring it until Sunday. How would I know today whether she was okay? Her breathing was so quiet and shallow there was no way I could listen for it above the sounds of the car engine and other highway noises. I sighed deeply and then carried on a conversation in my head, working through my fears.

"Okay, if she stops breathing, then what?" *You can pull over to the side of the highway.*

"And then what? Call 911?" *Calling 911 doesn't fit. They can't come and just hold your hand. If you call, you're asking them to intervene. That would be a painful disaster for all involved. You don't want EMTs pounding on her chest and cracking her ribs.*

"No, no. I don't want that." Heavy sigh.

"So then what?" *If you know she's dying, it will be tough to keep driving. You can't concentrate when you're bawling.*

"It would be nice to have a friend drive me so I can sit in the back with the baby. What if I called someone to bring us home?" *If you call somebody, how are you going to get the extra vehicle home? You can't leave a car unattended an hour's drive from home.*

"There's no help for it then. I will drive her home alone; she might pass away on the trip. God knows that's not how I want her to go, but I'm just going to have to deal with that possibility."

Once I finished talking to myself, I called out to Emmalynn, "You know what, baby girl? We have plans this evening. We are going to visit some friends. These women are excited to see you, and it would be great if you could just hang in there for a little while yet. . .please." I whispered softly, more as a prayer to Jesus than a request of Emmalynn.

Whether she understood on any level what I asked of her, I got in the car to drive.

Knowing I would be in Milwaukee, my friend Marie and I made plans to meet for supper to celebrate my upcoming birthday. We met at a hole-in-the-wall diner to hang out more than to enjoy the food. It was important to me that she meet Emmalynn.

During the last several years of my work as a bereavement specialist, Marie had been there to encourage me in my personal and professional life. She worked in the business office of the hospital where HALO was founded, and she had been my friend in good times and in bad, in sickness and in health. When I had wanted to give up during my extended illness, Marie had not given up hope and told me she was sure my days were not done yet. She knew I would rebound and would still be able to make a difference for babies and families who were facing death and the inevitable grief involved in the loss. Her emotional and spiritual support helped shine light into my darkest hours.

The mood during supper wasn't heavy. At one point I even joked, saying to Emmalynn, "Hey, little girl, just chill a moment, will ya?" as I put her in Marie's arms so I could use the restroom. This was an unnecessary admonishment, but I said it to lighten the mood and alleviate some of Marie's hesitation over being left to hold the baby while I was out of the room. I went out of my way to help ease tension regarding Emmalynn's physical state when others were around. This wasn't the first time Marie had been asked to step up to the plate and out of her comfort zone, and crazy enough, we're still friends.

I noted that Emmalynn still wasn't her normal self. I fed her again, and as the formula dripped through the tubing into her stomach, a thought flitted through my mind that this might be her last meal. I said good-bye to Marie and packed up the diaper bag again and rolled the oxygen tank out to the car.

I was happy about our plans for the evening, anticipating seeing some close friends whom I had bonded with in a grief recovery group. The women were part of the Elizabeth Ministry of St. Dominic Catholic Church. I wasn't there to bring Emmalynn as a show-and-tell item. Many of these caring women knew of my desire to care for terminally ill children and had supported me during my own health crisis. Yet they had never met this precious little baby, the fulfillment of my dream.

After placing Emmalynn and all her medical gear in the car once more, I headed to the meeting, which was being held at my friend Ann's home. I would reach between the front seats, stretching my arm back so my fingers could gently caress her cheek. She felt warm enough, and I hoped my touch would bring her the same comfort it brought me.

The sun had already set when I pulled into Ann's driveway. I honestly didn't know what I was going to see when I opened the door to the backseat. If Emmalynn was dead, I wouldn't crumble. I knew God would help me deal with whatever circumstances I had to face.

The tiny glowing bulb in the overhead lamp didn't give off much light. I leaned across the seat and looked carefully at Emmalynn. She was still breathing, though minimally. I took a deep breath of my own and told her, "Let's do this, girlfriend!"

I left the medical gear in the car, taking only Emmalynn and the car seat out. I walked into the side door of my friend Ann's home, hooking the car seat's handle in the crook of my arm. The porch light was on, welcoming me into a place I knew was filled with love. Ann and her husband, Bill, had raised nine children in this modest two-story home.

The twenty women of the Elizabeth Ministry were gathered in the living room. My friend Ann saw me enter and happily took charge of Emmalynn. I went back for the supplies. When I returned, I found Emmalynn had interrupted the planning meeting for the Sanctity of Human Life month. These ladies were of various ages and sizes, but all of them oohed and aahed over my little girl. I could tell that some of the women were itching to have a little baby in their embrace. Emmalynn complied, accepting the women's kisses and hugs without a peep of complaint.

These women knew Emmalynn embodied something sacred, something divinely ethereal that is not valued in our culture at large. The women were drawn together by a reverence for human life in any stage, and they would not dismiss Emmalynn just because of any malformations. Instead, she showed it was possible to be loved, to be known, and to be cared for in every way, even with such a bleak diagnosis. Seeing her eight-pound frame and recognizing her humanity in spite of her frail condition provided a reality check. She helped us understand in a whole new way that life—even with grand imperfections—is precious and should not only be protected but also be cherished.

Toward the end of the meeting, I pulled Emmalynn's little body onto my lap and turned her onto her tummy, laying her across my legs. I stroked her back with enough pressure to make it comforting and not a tickle. When I pulled her diaper down slightly to gently work my way down her spine, I could see her bum was slightly reddened from the pressure of sitting most of the day. It wasn't an open wound, but it pained me to see the skin was pinker than usual. I gently massaged the area, and even though I didn't cry in front of the women there, my heart was aching that she might have been uncomfortable.

When Emmalynn and I got home from the meeting, all five children were there, and Mark arrived home from work shortly afterward. I sat in the living room and attempted to feed Emmalynn, but the formula wouldn't slide down her nasogastric tube. This was a warning signal, and my suspicion that something was amiss was correct.

Andrew wondered what we were going to do if she couldn't eat.

"I think she's getting ready to go to heaven," I said. "She doesn't need to have formula if she's getting ready to go there."

I flushed Emmalynn's nighttime medications through her tube. Afterward she wasn't showing any signs of being Pentecostal at all, but I knew it was God and not the medicines at work.

I noticed that her arms and legs were cold and her skin

was mottled. This was further evidence that her body was shutting down. I wanted to do something to help her, and I'm not sure if I even formulated a coherent prayer at that time, but it occurred to me that I could share my body heat with her much like a mother kangaroo does while her baby is in the pouch.

I went upstairs and took off my own clothing, and put on my heavy, warm, fuzzy green bathrobe. When I got back downstairs to the dining room, Mark was singing to Emmalynn, holding her with her head tucked up under his chin. He knew I'd been told she was deaf, but he didn't care. He still talked to her and sang "Jesus Loves Me" as though she could hear every word. The vibration of Mark's voice through his throat soothed Emmalynn, and she was contentedly nestled in his embrace.

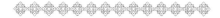

By 11:30 p.m. all the children kissed Emmalynn good-night and loved on her. One at a time each drifted off to bed. They all had things to do the next morning.

I was sitting in the chair at the dining room table, and Mark gazed at me. My normal bedtime would have been a few hours before, but he was taking my cue that things were different this night.

"Are you going to stay with her?" he asked.

"Yes, I am," I said quietly, nodding. "We'll see how it goes."

It was seventeen-year-old Charity's night to watch Emmalynn and sleep on the couch. She was ready for bed, wearing a T-shirt and shorts, her brown hair pulled back in a ponytail. She settled on the bench across the table, just a couple of feet from me. Mark said good night, and Charity and I were alone with our little girl. I believed the end was near; for a brief second I contemplated calling some hospice workers so I could hand Emmalynn over to professionals and have someone else shoulder the responsibility for knowing whether she was truly dying or not.

My prayers for her all along were that she would not die in the middle of the night lying in her little chair. I wanted her in my arms, close to me. I had the hospice phone number on the fridge, but I didn't call. I decided that this responsibility was one I wanted to bear myself.

I had taken off all of Emmalynn's clothing except for her tiny diaper and tucked her inside my bathrobe. She was lying on my chest, skin to skin, which is the best way to transfer heat to a baby who can't regulate temperature well on her own. My training as a nurse in the maternity ward was standing me in good stead now.

Emmalynn couldn't get any closer to my heart as her head rested on my breast. Her chest and tummy, arms and legs relaxed against my rib cage and abdomen. I could feel her melt against me, able to absorb the warmth of my skin into her own body. My bathrobe covered her backside, and my arms rested under her little bum to help hold her in place. She felt soft, quiet, and warm.

By this time, Emmalynn's breathing was shallow and infrequent. She wasn't in pain, the meds and my comfort measures had taken care of that. Miracle of miracles, she wasn't seizing either. I don't think she could have been more enveloped in love at that time.

I listened to her breath sounds as she began to "click," the sound a baby makes when breathing with only the top part of the lungs.

Close to midnight, Charity got up from the table where

she had been sitting with me. "I'm going to go lie down on the couch, okay? Call me if you need something." She was seventeen years old, but she had the presence of mind of a much older woman, and this was a solace to me.

I began to pray. Since I wasn't able to formulate anything coherent, it was more like, "Dear Jesus. Dear Jesus. Dear Jesus." I'm grateful God didn't need me to spell out in an eloquent way what my needs and desires were for my child. He knew what was most beneficial in that moment. I let Jesus be my go-between that night as Emmalynn and I sat with our hearts beating together as close as humanly possible.

Since I couldn't pray very well, I decided to sing "Jesus Loves Me." I had memorized the song as a young child and had repeated it over and over during times in my life when I was in so much pain I couldn't think straight. My voice was sputtering words between choked-back sobs. Not being able to hear probably helped Emmalynn to deal with my warbling.

Shortly after midnight I realized I had not heard Emmalynn "click" in the last minute or two. I opened my bathrobe and gently eased her away from my chest and looked down at her face. Her lips were white, and it was obvious that she was no longer with us. My stethoscope was sitting next to me on the table, and I picked it up to listen to her chest. I wanted to make sure she was indeed absent from her body.

I placed the stethoscope over her heart, but I couldn't hear anything except the rushing of my own blood.

In that moment I began to shudder, and gasping sobs overcame me. Hearing the change in my crying, Charity got up off the couch and hurried into the dining room. Her

T-shirt was rumpled and her ponytail askew.

"Is she gone?" she asked.

"I don't know for sure; I can't hear anything," I said, my voice shaking.

Charity took my stethoscope and placed it on Emmalynn's chest. "I don't hear a heartbeat," she said. Her eyes were red and tearful; she looked a little off balance. "What do we do now?"

And as quickly as the storm of my own weeping had come over me, it subsided.

"Go get your dad and the rest of the kids," I said. "We're going to be okay."

Charity went upstairs.

During those moments, I composed myself, gathering my wits. As a mom and a hospice nurse, I knew my kids would take their emotional cues from me, and I wanted to be ready. While grief was normal and struck the heart with a solid blow, Emmalynn's death was no reason to be filled with dread or panic. She had lived fifty days on earth. Now she would live an eternity in heaven.

My prevailing emotion was one of overwhelming gratitude that I had been able to love Emmalynn while she was passing. It was important that I had not been tense, that my heart rate had been steady. Emmalynn had not picked up any anxiety vibes from me. I had accomplished what I set out to do when she came to our home. Because of God's grace, I was able to stay steady when it was the most needed. I had wanted her to die in my embrace, being held by someone who loved her and knew her.

Over the years, I had grieved that Amie hadn't had human help close by when she died. That grief had motivated me to ask God for the strength and ability to do good and help others ease into the transition from this life to the next. I had helped lead Emmalynn to peace, and in the process I had discovered some of it too.

4

THE FUNERAL

To Thee, dear Lord, O Christ of God,
We sing, we ever sing;
Thou hast invaded death's abode
And robbed him of his sting.
The house of dust enthralls no more,
For Thou, the strong to save,
Thyself doth guard that silent door,
Great Keeper of the grave.

—ANNE ROSS COUSIN,
"TO THEE, DEAR LORD, O CHRIST OF GOD"

As our family gathered in the living room and adjoining areas, Mark came up behind me and quietly asked, "Is everybody okay here?" This was the first time our children had been this close to someone who died, especially a baby. I tried to reassure him, "I'm watching. They're doing great."

I placed Emmalynn in Mary Elisabeth's arms per her request. She held the baby and gently stroked the dimples in her hand formed by her tiny knuckles while chatting with Colette, one of the girls' friends. Colette sat on the carpet near Mary Elisabeth, and they were calmly conversing as though this were the most normal thing in the world.

I quietly called our hospice nurse and let her know

Emmalynn had passed into heaven. During my experience in working hospice, seeing the difference parents being calm can make in how their children coped emotionally, helped me now. While all of us were most certainly weeping at times, by grace no one was losing it.

Sometime after 2:00 a.m. the hospice nurse arrived, bringing with her our favorite social worker, Erin. Erin had been a gift to us during the time Emmalynn was living, and it was comforting to me that she made the extra effort to come be with us in the middle of the night.

Erin sat down on the living room floor with eleven-year-old Emily and asked how she was doing. They played a game of cards and chatted together for a little bit while I worked with the hospice nurse to complete paperwork at the kitchen counter. Erin wandered back into the dining area and said with conviction, "This is how it's supposed to be."

I nodded in agreement. The way our family was responding to Emmalynn's death was truly a gift from God.

We all sat, waiting for the coroner. He's a huge man, burly and bearlike. While I was a hospital nurse, I'd had interactions with him, and I knew that anytime after midnight is not his favorite time of day. Let's just say his people skills can be lacking when they are most needed in the wee hours of the morning.

I was a little fearful the coroner would be gruff and ornery, and my Jesus knew I didn't want to cope with that. When he came through the front door at 3:00 a.m., he asked about the Christmas lights that were lit up on the porch. "It's my idea so first responders can find our house easily," I acknowledged, wondering if I was going to get grief about it. Instead, he said, "I like it!"

The coroner spent a few minutes with the nurse, signing his name in the right places. He checked Baby Emmalynn and then came over to the end of our dining room table where I was seated. I was braced for some negative fallout. But he unexpectedly put his big hand on my shoulder and squeezed it gently. "You did good," was all he said. The affirmation was a balm to my soul, and remembering that moment can still make tears smart in my eyes.

I called the funeral home myself and let the director know Emmalynn had died. He asked if I wanted him to come get her.

"Are you out and about at this hour?" I responded.

He laughed and said, "Not hardly."

"Then we'll bring her in the morning," I said. "We need to get squared away here at the house. We can get plans figured out then."

The nurse, social worker, coroner, and Colette left to go home.

Once again the family was ready to go off to bed, this time for the rest of the night. Charity piped up, "I'll stay with Emmalynn. It was my night anyway."

Mark looked at me in disbelief, but I could tell he was impressed with Charity's maturity. He had been concerned that taking in a baby with a terminal diagnosis would prove to be detrimental to our family's emotional health. While Emmalynn's needs had sometimes been a source of tension and anxiety, the benefits of caring for her *far* outweighed any negative consequences.

I went upstairs but was unable to sleep, tossing restlessly. I softly crept back down the stairs and to the living room to find Emmalynn snuggled into her recliner as usual. Charity was on the couch next to her, lying on her tummy, with her arm stretched out toward Emmalynn. Charity's hand was gently resting on top of the Winnie the Poo baby blanket. Charity had slightly curled Emmalynn's little left fist around her finger one last time before falling asleep.

I sat down on the floor on the other side of Emmalynn and curled her right hand over my finger. I couldn't really pray in that moment, but I was reflective. The Bible says that Jesus' mother Mary was told about the forthcoming baby and "kept all these things, and pondered them in her heart" (Luke 2:19 kjv). I sat next to Emmalynn in the early morning hours and pondered too.

When Mark came down about 6:30 a.m. to get the day started, I went back upstairs to my bedroom to get a little rest.

I later learned that when Andrew came to the kitchen for breakfast he was a bit wild-eyed. "Where's the baby?" he asked with a little anxiety.

"Emmalynn is in the living room with Charity," Mark assured him.

Andrew went into the living room and pulled his baby sister into his arms. He held her carefully and kissed her and cried and said good-bye. Then he finished getting ready and went off to school.

For months I had no idea how important it was my son had this time with Emmalynn.

I got up for the day about 9:30 a.m.

"Mom," Charity said, "Emmalynn has kind of thrown up on her sleeper and blanket, and she's stiff."

"I know, sweetheart," I said. "I'll take care of her."

I hugged my brave kiddo who was finding her way through all of this with a somber uncertainty but determined to be part of it all.

I pulled together what was needed for the funeral home and gathered Emmalynn into my arms for the last time and carried her precious little body out to the car. Mark drove while I sat in the passenger's seat holding my baby. Charity was in the back, along to help in whatever way necessary. She was embracing all the aspects of caring for a dying child from start to finish.

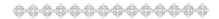

Emmalynn's funeral was scheduled for a Monday morning. It was an inconvenient time for family and friends to attend, but I wasn't able to arrange a better one. A small stipend through Medicaid covered the cost of the casket, embalming, and the opening and closing of the grave. The burial site itself was gifted to us as was the time donated by the funeral home personnel. With all the medical debt we had acquired over the course of my most recent illnesses and surgeries, we had little money to pay for anything grander than the bare basics.

I was surprised at how foggy my thinking was after Emmalynn died. I had thought the shock of her death would leave me numb but able to function. This wasn't the case. I had to make decisions about where she should be buried, which pink sleeper she should wear, which knitted hat, and what blanket to wrap her in. That I would never see her or those items again was cause for an almost continual flood of tears. Honestly, how can a body produce so much moisture? I have no clue how I didn't end up completely dehydrated given the volume of water flowing from my eyes and cascading down my cheeks.

I woke up on Monday, the day of Emmalynn's funeral, and could hardly move. My body felt as if it weighed a thousand pounds. I was dreading going to the service. How silly it seemed to have called it a celebration while planning for it the week before.

The tears wouldn't quit flowing.

I didn't know what I was going to wear. I wasn't sure anyone was going to be there because several people had told me they couldn't get the time off work to attend or they simply couldn't bring themselves to come because they felt it too sad.

I lay in bed until 9:20 a.m. when my husband finally said to me with concern but gentleness, "You're going to go to the funeral, right? I mean, we need to leave in a few minutes and you're not even dressed?" That man is a saint. Not once did he say, "You know, we never should have done this. I don't want you crying. That's it! We're not doing this again. I had no idea you'd take it this hard. I'm sorry I agreed."

That would have made me angry and feeling guilty for mourning. Emmalynn was deeply loved, and our grief over her death was legitimate and mirrored the emotional investment we had made.

I struggled to get out of bed and stood in front of the mirror in the bathroom. I sternly told myself repeatedly, "You've got to stop bawling!" I didn't listen very well, and that was evidenced by the blotchy face, the swollen eyelids, and the inability to apply any makeup because my tears would have washed it right off again in streaks.

Choosing clothing from my closet and getting dressed was like trying to run in a swimming pool; every movement was labored and more work than I felt I could manage.

I put on a simple white blouse with thin pink-and-black stripes and a black skirt. I looked like death wearing all black, the traditional funeral color, but no one needed to wonder any more than they already would be, if I would have the strength to remain standing.

We pulled up to the funeral home, and oh my goodness, you have no idea how wonderful it was to see the folks who made the effort to attend. I felt my heart lighten up a little to see the faces and feel the hugs people offered. No one spoke unkind words, stating some version of "She wasn't your real kid. What are you so sad for?"

Instead, as one of my friends put it, "We tried to hold back as though to guard ourselves from being hurt, but instead, we caved and fell in love with Emmalynn."

Given Emmalynn was a baby, we had expected attendance to be nominal and set up only a couple dozen chairs. I mean, how many friends does a fifty-day-old little girl have? Well, she had enough that three adjoining rooms were filled and we ran out of folders.

My son, Andrew, bless his heart, is a natural host. He took the memorial folders and handed them out and helped people find a seat and sign the guest book. He was not paid staff that day but fell into the role easily and made those who came feel welcome and wanted.

A few weeks before Emmalynn died, I had asked John, our worship pastor at Crossroads Community Church, to officiate at her service. He had looked a little taken aback when I requested his help. I told him to think about it and let me know. When Pastor John followed up on my request, he said he would be happy to play his guitar, sing, and help give the sermon at the funeral. I didn't find out until after Emmalynn's service was concluded that not only was her service the first child's funeral he had officiated, but it was also his first funeral, period. He stepped up, creating a wonderful memory even though he had the unenviable task of giving the parting message for a child.

During Emmalynn's service, the attendees had the opportunity to share a memory of her or one way she'd had an impact on their lives. Jonathan, our eldest son, stood up and shared with the group first.

> "I questioned if bringing Emmalynn home was
> the best idea, knowing her condition was terminal.
> Was it worth getting to know, care for her, and
> love her only to see her go so soon? And my mom
> said that she'd rather have her die at home with
> people who cared for her than in the hospital.
> After she came and went, I couldn't agree more. It
> made us stronger as a family."

My son Joshua spoke after his brother. He told everyone he hadn't wanted to come home from college after Emmalynn had been brought home. He had been concerned, really concerned. "Ah, Mom," he said, "what are you doing?! Haven't we been through enough already without adding this too?" He was referring to the serious negative outcomes of my surgeries and autoimmune disasters. Why in the world was I choosing to bring a terminally ill baby home to die? It made no human sense to him. These were his words regarding our family: "We'd been in survival mode, barely existing for a couple of years." We had experienced so much unbelievable loss on every front.

But to Joshua's surprise and relief, once he had decided to come home and meet our little darling, he was amazed at the transformation in our home. He said, "Where it had been just black and white, all of a sudden there was color—everywhere."

Mary Elisabeth shared next. She had pulled night duty with her little sister. She has always worked very hard to keep up with her next oldest sisters. Both Johanna and Charity handled the night shift with Emmalynn. Mary Elisabeth wasn't really feeling super brave, but not to be outdone or left in the dust, she also helped shoulder the burden. She was honest with folks:

"I just remember at one point not being sure if she was breathing or not because it was raspy. So I turned the light back on and rocked her in her seat and decided I'd stay up with her until she died or relaxed. I think that's when I decided that she would not be alone while I tried to sleep. I talked to her a lot too, until I eventually fell asleep. I was a bit scared of her dying while I was on shift, but I gave it up to God, and there was great peace in that, and I stopped being scared of Emmalynn's condition so much.

It was a good opportunity to grow and to pray. In those situations, you learn to trust in God's sovereignty more than ever. It was comforting and necessary that my mom told us it wasn't our fault if she died, and that if we needed anything she was right down the hall. It took the pressure off from external sources. But there's always internal pressure not to mess up in case you're the one to cause her death. I guess I just figured she was worth it."

A number of women gave testimony of how this tiny little girl had affected their lives. For some of the mothers, she was the first baby they had held since their own had died. The healing she brought to hearts ravaged by grief over their own previous losses was a completely unexpected blessing of sharing her little self with our friends. Stan and Bess both came to her services and expressed the redemption they felt over the loss of their beloved son, Davey, who hadn't been granted the dignity of a funeral. They believed God was answering their prayers and healing their grief through Emmalynn's life and death.

The most amazing realization I expressed that morning was that Emmalynn needed me in my weakness. She didn't need me busy. She couldn't maintain her temperature well, so we held her almost constantly to keep her warm. I could do lots of cuddling while sitting or lying down. She didn't really need me to *do* much for her but simply to *be* with her. She was most in need of being loved, and this I could do whether I was physically strong or not.

Daniel, my sweet young friend who has not let Down syndrome define him and dictate what he can and cannot do, wrote and shared this poem about Emmalynn:

All is calm,
all is bright outside tonight.
In this moment of silence
I am on my own.
I'm standing still in the memory of Emmalynn,
my dearest, sweetest friend.
We are letting her go home.
She is in His hands.
In tears we're rejoicing.

No meal was planned for after the funeral so that folks could stay and mingle, and they couldn't have anyway because they needed to go about their Monday-morning business. After we said good-bye to those who came to support us, I had a sense of *What now?*

Our family went back to the house, which was strangely quiet since the oxygen concentrator had stopped its rhythmic humming and pulsing. Emmalynn's recliner was in the living room on the floor. Her oxygen tubing was strewn about, her medical paraphernalia shouting to all who looked that our baby had certainly existed, lived, and breathed but now was gone. I couldn't do anything with her things. I could not clean them up or throw them away.

I did make one phone call to a couple from church, Jesse and Taylor. They are like younger siblings to me. I asked them to please wash Emmalynn's car seat and the stroller so I could put them away clean. Emmalynn had spit up, and her formula had leaked out onto the fabric. I had no mental reserve left to remove and wash and reinstall the coverings.

Taylor came over and picked up the car seat and stroller combo. He stood in our entryway and couldn't stop the tears. He asked Emily, "Are you okay? I don't know how you did this."

Emily looked up at him and said, "We helped her to have a life before she died. It was a good thing, and I'm glad we could do it for her." This simple statement made the big man cry all the harder.

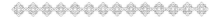

One of my girlfriends had given me a gift card for my birthday, which was the day after Emmalynn died. I had spent my birthday going over funeral details with Pastor John, so I hadn't really done any celebrating. I wasn't in any mood to do it anyway.

Now that the funeral was over, I made the decision to take the gift card to one of my favorite restaurants and go have some lunch by myself. Field to Fork was emptying out because it was nearly 1:00 in the afternoon. I had brought a book to read, asked for a table in the corner, and tucked myself as far away from people as possible. I don't even remember what book it was and didn't accomplish much reading. I sat and contemplated all that had taken place and watched those milling around me. Forks were clanking against plates, glasses clinking in the sink where the kitchen help was washing them, voices calling loudly, "Your order's up!" General hustle and bustle filled the restaurant, and no one in the room had a clue my baby was being carried to the cemetery and being buried as they sat in their seats, normal lives appearing to go on without a hiccup. No thought given to the mother in the corner grieving the death of her child while others fussed about their food being too hot or too cold or their child not winning his basketball game. The fact the world did not stop spinning for even a second for anyone else, not even me, left me feeling incredulous. How many people do I see in a day who have just had a major loss in their lives and I walk past and don't see them at all and don't recognize they are in pain?

After lunch I drove to the cemetery. I had been told Emmalynn would be placed in the infant section, and I knew where that was. I slowly came around the circle to the left and was momentarily confused. I didn't see a mound of earth to mark her grave. On closer inspection, I realized a small rectangle of sod had been placed over the grave that held Emmalynn's casket, and two wilted roses were lying on top. We hadn't even had the presence of mind to order flowers for the funeral, and though one other family, friends of Jonathan's, had thought of sending a bouquet, a mix-up at the flower shop kept the flowers from being delivered. The two limp roses, almost colorless against the dried, matted, faded green grass could easily have been missed had I not been searching for evidence they were there. This cut me to the core.

No stone. No large display of flowers, just a chunk of dirt and grass removed and placed back almost as though the grave didn't exist.

But it did exist. There was a grave.

A new one.

A baby was in that tiny white casket.

My baby was in that grave.

For a few seconds, I fought waves of nausea. I panicked, thinking, *I can't leave her here. It's dark. She's alone. She'll be cold. Oh God*, I groaned, *this is too much to bear. I can't. I can't!*

For the first time ever, I understood the scene in *Gone with the Wind* when Rhett Butler refused to allow his daughter, Bonnie, to be buried.

The intensity of my grief shredded any semblance of control I might have exercised earlier in the day. I understood from a practical standpoint that even if I did dig up the dirt again and move it aside, I could not and should not bring her casket out of there and home. But I still had to work through my thoughts in my usual way.

"If you got out of the car and dug up the casket, then what?" *You can't change that she died.*

"So now what?" *You cannot change that this is the way it goes. Bodies are buried or cremated or lost on earth in some other fashion. That's the reality, woman, smack-you-in-the-face reality, but you're going to have to deal with your helplessness here.*

I felt as though I could not breathe, the sorrow and loss were so overwhelming. Just my Jesus and me, working it through. And faithful as always, He answered my prayer in a completely unexpected but absolutely appropriate and soul-touching way. He was touched by my grief and He was weeping with me, but not because He was helpless to do anything for me.

I was still sitting in the car, with the engine running, on the paved driveway that was only a few feet from the infant section and Emmalynn's grave.

At that precise moment a song by Gungor came on the radio, "You make beautiful things out of the dust. . ." From dust we came and to dust we will return. Emmalynn was not in the grave, but her little body was being cradled in God's creation of earth. Her body would eventually be resurrected—beautifully whole and well.

I remembered a scene from the book *Faith Like Potatoes*. It tells the story of a four-year-old boy named Alistair who is run over by a tractor driven by his uncle Angus. The grief tears Angus apart, and he explains:

> I was racked by guilt, and couldn't eat or sleep. The nights were the worst. . . . Every time I closed my eyes, I felt the jolt of the tractor. . .[and] saw Alistair's little body lying limply in my arms.
>
> The devil was quick to accuse me. The thoughts went round in my head day and night: "You killed your brother's son! It was your negligence that killed him. You should have been more careful. You're not worthy to be a witness for Jesus."[1]

In a dream Alistair's father, Fergus, sees his son running toward him through emerald-green fields. Fergus catches the boy up in his strong arms and swings him around in the air while they laugh together. Fergus asks his son if he wants to come back, and Alistair answers, "No, Dad, I'm waiting for you."

Even though it's the middle of the night, Fergus calls Angus and shares the vision he had with his brother, helping to assuage the guilt and the grief Angus had been experiencing. Angus writes:

> "I know that eternity is real. When I reach the pearly gates through the grace of God, there is going to be a little boy named Alistair waiting for me, and we will recognise each other. . . . As I grew in Jesus through this experience, I came to realise that life is nothing but a vapor, a puff of smoke that soon blows away. Our real eternal life is safe in the hands of God."[2]

If I could call to Emmalynn and ask if she wanted to come back, she would say, "No, Mommy, I'm waiting for you in heaven, and I can't wait to show it to you!"

Logically, all this agonizing pain and grief could have been completely avoided. We did have that choice. But we had also received so much joy because of her little life, which we would never have known had we shielded ourselves from the hurt.

My feelings became less desperate and out of control. God promises a peace that passes understanding, and thankfully He quieted my soul. The cemetery situation was not without any tangible ways to make it more bearable, and I was gifted with the ability to sort through the troubles in my head and also think, *What* can *you change?*

The pathetic flowers on Emmalynn's grave made me sad. I opened the car door, stepped over the curb onto the grass, and stooped down. I picked up the wilted stems, walked back across the road, and threw them in the trash can. Getting back in the car, I promised Emmalynn, "I'll be right back, baby."

I then went to see my sweet friend Maggie at the monument store. I told her, "I need something to mark Emmalynn's grave until her headstone is finished. Please help me."

Maggie took me over to where there was a grave marker with the face of an angel and the words "In the arms of the angels far away from here" written on it. It was perfect to mark the spot until her own stone could be crafted. I took the grave marker to the cemetery and gently placed it on the small patch of sod.

One of the verses I had chosen for HALO was Matthew 18:10: "See that you do not despise one of these little ones. For I tell you that their angels in heaven always see the face of my Father in heaven" (NIV). I had shared this comforting verse with many of the families I helped during my time as a bereavement specialist. Our babies were not lost, wandering about or ceasing to exist entirely. They could no longer be in our arms, but they were in someone's arms; their own angels in heaven held them for the time being. I was living what I had been sharing with others for years and finding it enough in the throes of bearing my own grief.

5

FLAWS REVEALED AND HEALED

Grace, grace, God's grace,
Grace that will pardon and cleanse within;
Grace, grace, God's grace,
Grace that is greater than all our sin!

—Julia H. Johnston,
"Grace Greater Than Our Sin"

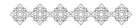

This line by *Downton Abbey*'s Lord Grantham to his butler has recently made it into our cultural lexicon: "My dear fellow, we all have chapters we would rather keep unpublished."[1] Well, these next two are a couple of mine.

I have heard, "I love you so much!" time and time again from people who have read what my family and I do in caring for terminally ill kiddos. I appreciate it, really I do!

But it's also superficial.

It's abundantly more meaningful to me when folks know me well—flaws highlighted—and they still stick around.

Tim Keller profoundly sums up my feeling:

"To be loved but not known is comforting but superficial. To be known and not loved is our greatest fear. But to be fully known and truly loved is, well, a lot like being loved by God. It is what we need more than anything. It liberates us from pretense, humbles us out of our self-righteousness, and fortifies us for any difficulty life can throw at us."[2]

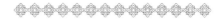

While Emmalynn was living with us, Mark and I began the licensing paperwork to become medical-treatment foster parents because that was the best way to be in a position to receive a Safe Haven baby. We especially wanted those who were born with a lethal anomaly or a terminal diagnosis whose parents could not deal with it and had safely relinquished the child to authorities. This child would not have dozens of people lining up to take him or her home but rather would need a family like ours ready to do hospice care. After Emmalynn's funeral, our family was most assuredly still grieving, but our sorrow over her passing had not incapacitated us. The social worker in charge of the process had left us alone to grieve for a few weeks. One day I summoned the mental energy to call and ask her what was next. She informed me that a social worker from the foster care agency would visit our home. I knew she was to meet with and interview each of my children privately, and I didn't have a clue what she would ask or how they would respond.

After the social worker met with Andrew, she pulled me aside and said, "I asked Andrew if he wanted to take in another baby who was going to die. He said, 'I don't want to do it. It was too scary.'" She said she had not promised Andrew it wouldn't happen again and suggested that I talk to him about it.

I took this advice to heart because I was not purposely trying to traumatize any of my children. Before discussing the conversation with Andrew, I spent time praying. One morning on the way to school, I casually asked him, "You told the social worker having Emmalynn was too scary. Can you tell me what bothered you?"

He sighed. "I never knew when she was going to die," he said. "And I was afraid when I went to school that she would die and I wouldn't know. I might come home and find she was gone. I don't want to do that."

I asked hesitantly, "So you weren't scared she was going to die; you were afraid because you weren't going to be there?"

He nodded. "Yes, I want to be there if I can. I don't want them to be gone and not be able to see them again."

Feeling my way tentatively, trying not to assume or put words in his mouth, I asked, "If we get another baby who is terminal, if and when that might ever happen, when they die, if I promise to come and get you wherever you might be at the time and bring you home and let you see the baby and say good-bye, are you good with that?"

"Yeah, totally." Then, in his typical middle school fashion, he said, "Hey, Mom! I've been thinking about teleportation. Like I could make a car that you could just get in it and think about where you wanted to go and it would go. You wouldn't even have to drive it yourself! Wouldn't that be cool?"

"Uh, yes," I answered. "Sure, that'd be cool."

Apparently the subject of having more hospice kiddos had been resolved and we had moved on to the next thing.

I dropped Andrew off at school, and I pulled over at the cemetery on the way back home. I gave myself a moment to weep with gratefulness for the outcome of our conversation. I'd had no idea my boy was struggling with the possibility he might not be there when Emmalynn died.

The decision to keep Emmalynn with us through the night—though I was in the dark about Andrew's fears and his desire for closure—was an affirmation from God to him and me.

In late October 2012, we completed our medical treatment foster parent education requirements, but more in-depth background checks would take weeks to complete. Over Thanksgiving I sent an email message to the social worker asking whether everything in the licensing process had been wrapped up.

In reply I received a cryptic email saying there were some glitches that we would have to address. I swallowed a lump in my throat and wondered what they could be. The second week of December, Mark and I sat in our living room as the social worker told us we had some serious issues to deal with. Both Mark and I took deep breaths, or maybe held them, thinking, *Good grief, what's up now?*

The social worker asked about a 1999 incident when the police had pulled Mark over. He had been riding a motorcycle along with four-year-old Charity, who was on the front of the bike. The helmet on her head was so heavy her neck couldn't hold the weight, so she was riding with her head tilted onto Mark's forearm as they cruised slowly around the block.

The policeman warned Mark that it wasn't safe for her to be in the front and that she should be riding behind him. The officer didn't issue a ticket, and Mark never told me about the incident, so I was surprised upon hearing about it now. Mark was irritated that something like that would even be considered a concern. The news was a little disconcerting to say the least.

But the social worker wasn't done.

She looked down at the papers in her hand and then up at me. She hesitated, shrugging her shoulders, as if to say that this had to be addressed whether it was comfortable or not. "Cori," she said, "your record shows a chapter 51 in 2010 that you didn't tell me about." She was not harsh with me and said sympathetically, "It looks like you were trying to hide it, and not disclosing it is worse than telling me about it in the first place."

I felt as though all the air had been sucked out of the room.

I had no idea that my brief stay in a psych ward was on my record, because I had been told it had never been made an official incident in my health history. I had never gone to court for it. The foster care application had not asked a direct question about it. I had no intention of hiding anything; I honestly hadn't known the "almost" chapter 51 filing was a problem. The filing applies if a physician determines the patient is "dangerous" and "evidences a substantial probability of physical harm to himself or herself as manifested by evidence of recent threats of or attempts at suicide or serious bodily harm."[3]

A huge wave of shame washed over me. My heart was racing, my gut rolling, my palms sweating. All the reasons in the world why I was the biggest loser on the planet careened around in my head. Who was I to think I should be a foster parent? The past is not supposed to define your present, but sometimes it does. When you put a nail in a wall, you leave a hole. Our actions have consequences that can be forgiven but not necessarily forgotten.

I stammered through a difficult explanation about a

period of depression, wondering if "Me thinks thou doth protest too much" was the way the social worker perceived my ramblings. Our culture isn't friendly to people who fail. At the end of a football game, I might comment on the losing players, "Oh, those poor guys. They really tried hard." My compassion for the unsuccessful team is not necessarily shared by my friends and family members. My sentiments are usually met with a harsher viewpoint: "They lost, Cori. They lost. It doesn't matter if they tried."

I wasn't sure if my explanation was going to be adequate or whether a desperate choice in my past would define my life and limit my ability to do what I desired.

The social service worker said the chapter 51 would not necessarily disqualify me, but I would have to undergo a psych evaluation.

After the social worker stood, gathered her papers, and left our home, I told Mark, "We don't have to do this. They need all our financial information. They want to talk to all of our kids without us in the room. They want personal history from our childhoods. This is incredibly intrusive to have people we don't know combing through our lives and making decisions about our worthiness to foster. We do not have to do this."

It was enough that I was ashamed of myself. I didn't want Mark to feel compelled to go through the process. He doesn't think it's anybody's business what he ate for lunch yesterday let alone all the in-depth information required to get licensed. I was surprised but steadied and encouraged by his response. "We're not going to quit," he said. "They can look at all our stuff and tell us they don't want us, but we're not going to walk away until we get licensed or it's impossible to move forward."

God knew bringing Emmalynn into our lives first, with applying to be foster parents second, was the way He would fortify us to have the wherewithal to put our fears of being rejected aside and continue to pursue the capability of caring for another child in a similar situation. The experience with Emmalynn made it totally worth the hassle!

For forty-six years, my GI issues had severely limited my ability to psychologically cope. Since my body was not contributing in any positive way to my being able to deal with life's difficulties, God's grace in preserving me all that time was now evident to me. However, there was a time when all I could see was what was wrong and hurting and broken. My church background led me to believe I was supposed to prosper if I was doing the right thing. Somehow God's end of the bargain was to make life doable for me if I obeyed His rules. Now, on one level, this is accurate. Discipline and punishment don't have to be meted out if you walk the straight and narrow. But we're also promised there will be trouble in this life. Suffering is to be expected; it's not an unusual occurrence.

My immature perspective of suffering compelled me to share with God that I did not do hard. I was not a soldier. I also had no desire to become one, thank you very much. I wanted to have struggles and suffering that were manageable. I wanted to run from trouble as fast and as far away as possible or get through it quickly and move on to what I considered better things.

It is pathetic that I told Jesus that I didn't know why He caused or allowed tough things in my life because I prayed to Him and liked Him much better when things were going well. Didn't He want me to like Him?

Even more serious was the spiritual deal I had laid on

the table as early as my teen years. If things got too hard and I couldn't handle it, I was "out of here." I reserved the right to decide when I'd had enough and that I would have a say in the timing of my departure to heaven. I knew Jesus as my Savior. I was not afraid of death. I was more afraid of not living successfully, of being sick and disabled, and of feeling as though I was more trouble than I was worth to my family and friends. What a shaky, miserable place to stand. All around me were pits of emotional quicksand ready to pull me under based on my faulty estimations of my value and my ability to carry on under great duress.

Throughout my entire life I had struggled with being ill. Having recurring incapacitating pain was a cross I did not want to bear. While suffering for Jesus on the mission field was supposedly virtuous, having intestinal spasms that left me lying on the floor wasn't considered spiritual at all! In fact, a lot of people told me it was my fault—I must be doing something wrong.

Reading an essay by biblical counselor Dr. David Powlison strangely comforted my heart as I resonated with his words.

> "Suffering often brings a doubled pain. In the first place there is "the problem" itself—sickness, poverty, betrayal, bereavement. That is hard enough (and this promise speaks comfort). But it is often compounded by a second problem. Other people, even well-meaning, often don't respond very well to sufferers. Sufferers are often misunderstood, or meddled with, or ignored. . . .
>
> Faulty diagnoses, misguided treatments, negative side effects, contradictory advice, huge

waste of time and money, false hopes repeatedly dashed, false fears pointlessly rehearsed, no plausible explanation forthcoming, blaming the victim, and declining sympathy as compassion fatigue sets in for would-be helpers!"[4]

I have been a "problem" person ever since I can remember. At birth I had to contend with congenital nephritis, and the cause was never found. My mother tells me the doctors cut me in half from belly button to back bone and did a kidney biopsy. I still bear the long scar.

As a child, I also had frequent bouts with sore throats and respiratory infections to the point where I would be coughing up blood. These episodes resulted in multiple treatments with antibiotics. (The drug of choice at the time was tetracycline, and it discolored my teeth, causing them to turn gray.) After all the antibiotic treatment for infections I consumed, it's no wonder I had GI issues.

When I was fourteen, I attended a camp in New Mexico where the boys found it greatly entertaining to throw cow pies into the drainage ditch where we girls brushed our teeth and bathed. I picked up amoebic dysentery and was so dreadfully ill that I lost fifteen pounds in a week. With only eighty-five pounds left on my five-foot-three frame, I was skin and bones. I didn't learn until nursing school that the lack of fat on my body left me with no estrogen stores to have a period until I was back up to a more normal weight.

When my cycles started back up—O help me, Jesus—they came back with a vengeance. Every month for two to three days, I would be on the floor, curled up in a ball, experiencing the worst cramping, vomiting, diarrhea, and fainting I had ever had.

My system was in a constant state of inflammation, and doctors found it tricky to pinpoint where it had gone awry. The medications, procedures, surgeries, and ER visits to treat symptoms of an ever-widening array of troubles were expensive and humiliating.

In the fall of my senior year of college, I was hospitalized twice. The root cause of my pain was unknown and attributed to stress. I struggled with despair. How could I be feeling this badly and functioning so poorly and yet not have a diagnosis? My pain was constant because every day I was eating foods that my body couldn't handle, but I did not know this, and neither did any of the physicians who attempted to treat me. I couldn't seem to keep up with the demands of school and work, and some of my college advisers told me others coped much better with the same stress, so what was my problem? I didn't have a clue.

I heard several comments from well-meaning (and not-so-well-meaning) friends and classmates: "You know, maybe God has to hit you upside the head with a two-by-four in order to knock some sense into you." Pastors advised me to repent of my unconfessed sin so I could be healed of my many maladies. I felt angry and bewildered and wondered what I was doing that was so evil I had to be punished.

Confused, I let their comments create a deep sense of despair in my soul. Carrying on day after day feeling as though I had been singled out for punishment was difficult, and I was at a loss as to what exactly I should do to fix myself so God could bless me—blessing being equated with good health, good grades, and a happy life in general.

My nursing instructors were also bewildered and were concerned about my health, absences, and fragile mental state. In November 1987, just weeks away from graduation, my psych instructor advised me to withdraw from the nursing program because she did not see me passing the rotation.

Not passing? The news devastated me. I had never failed anything in my life. My identity was wrapped up in getting excellent grades and being at the top of my class. In anything that had to do with sheer will, natural talent, or hard work, I wasn't lacking.

One night shortly after I withdrew from the nursing program, I lay in bed, drenching my pillow with tears. I felt desperate and unproductive and as if I were a liability to everyone. I made sweeping judgments about others' perceptions of me, which weren't accurate but reflected my feelings at the time. I whispered to no one in particular, "Could somebody just love me for me?"

God's answer was swift and sure, indelibly pressed on my heart and mind, though I did not hear an audible voice. He communicated, *I loved you before you were born, before you'd ever done anything good or bad. My love is not dependent on your ability to perform.*

I reenrolled in nursing school in January 1988, and when I arrived to register, I was asked to step aside and speak with the financial adviser. I stood there waiting to hear what he had to say, trembling. I imagined I would hear that I was a failure. What was I doing trying to come back again? I prayed, silent and deep, *Dear God, I believe I should finish. I started this course to become a nurse. I can't just quit. So, You make it possible to get this done.*

The financial guy beckoned me to sit near him, and even though it was winter and chilly, I was sweating bullets waiting to hear what he would say.

"I see here you were enrolled in your last semester of nursing school this past fall, right?" he asked.

I nodded.

"Okay, well, I also see you paid for your semester even though you didn't finish it. You were hospitalized a couple of times too?" He wasn't callously probing but rather compassionately inquiring.

I nodded affirmatively again, thinking it was all over my record that I couldn't cope well with my physical ailments or with the school load.

Instead, he looked back at his computer screen and told me with a smile, "You know, I think it's great you're back again! I'm going to transfer the monetary credits from last semester to this one. You've already got your books, and along with the Pell grant for this semester, you're good to go. Finish well!"

I was speechless, having no idea God could answer my prayers over and abundantly above all I could ask or think. I graduated without difficulty and with great grades on May 21, 1988.

I got married a week later.

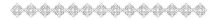

Almost four years earlier, in August 1984, the lyrics from a Roberta Flack song—"The First Time Ever I Saw Your Face"—came true for me: I thought "the sun rose" in someone's eyes. That day the sun was streaming through the high windows as we waited to register for our classes in the hallway of the Old Main building at Maranatha Baptist Bible College just west of Madison. I turned my head and caught sight of Mark standing a little farther down the line. His hair was blond with natural curl and shine. His eyes were bright blue, and he smiled at me.

"Be still my heart" hardly cut it. The pump in my chest nearly stopped.

I instantly thought, *Oh my goodness, you're going to marry that guy.* Then I faced away quickly, berating myself for being so silly. *You're only eighteen years old. You just got here. You've got four years of school to finish. Good grief, you don't even know his name or whether he's already married.*

A few weeks after that fateful encounter, Mark and I were in Speech 101 class. As part of our coursework, we students were told to prepare personal testimonies to share with the other students. On the day it was Mark's turn, he stood and said he was twenty-nine years old and fresh out of the Air Force. (I wanted to do a jig in my seat, and was singing the "Hallelujah Chorus" in my head upon hearing his age. I thought all college freshmen were eighteen years old and dumb as a box of rocks. Not so!) Even more impressive than his age was his desire to learn more about God and his willingness to become a missionary. He expressed with an endearing earnestness that his salvation and loving Jesus were the most important things in his life. I was moved to tears with joy.

How could it get any better than that?!

I shared my testimony the next week, mentioning the time I had spent on the Navajo reservation in New Mexico, but I didn't share my specific desire to serve in India. I confess that part of the reason I remained mum about India was because I wasn't sure where Mark thought he wanted to go, and I was leaving my options open.

After class as I walked past him in chapel, he called out, "Speech! Speech!" to me. I thought it was pretty sweet he had paid any attention. I effortlessly chatted with him and decided to ask, "So, you mentioned you wanted to be a missionary. Where?"

Mark replied, "Oh, India, I think."

I was dumbfounded and even more convinced this guy was going to marry me someday.

I responded with, "You know, that's where I've thought about going, too."

I later learned that Mark shared our conversation with his dorm buddies and they hooted and hollered. They said, "Ha, you could've said you wanted to go to Timbuktu, and she'd have said that was her mission field too. *Bahahaha!*"

Oh, I was mad. I wanted to go to India long before those dumb guys assumed it was a ploy to get Mark's attention!

Mark told me not long after we met as freshman that I was a buxom babe, and he liked that. In other words, I had packed on the "freshman fifteen," but he didn't mind the way I had left the teenybopper figure behind for a more womanly shape. We didn't really date but rather had many lively discussions in the snack room in the basement of the college. We also found many reasons to argue, and while he said he liked my fiery spirit, he didn't have time to tame a young filly. "Find yourself a young buck and have a bunch of fat babies" was his admonition time and again during our college days.

Mark was steadfast in his determination to be the next apostle Paul, a celibate preacher and martyr. Women, he explained, were a distraction, and he was not altogether happy to find that this Baptist college housed hundreds of women when he had expected a men-only kind of seminary setting. (His expectation was based on his Catholic background and the fact the college had been a monastery at one time.)

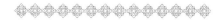

In my sophomore year, I started the nursing program at Madison Area Technical College that partnered with Maranatha Baptist. Mark and I saw each other only occasionally at church.

During this year of nursing school, I was hospitalized a couple of times when my period set off intense spasms in my large intestine, which would result in my passing out on the floor. This hormone-induced spasming did not show up on CT scans or in blood work or in the invasive exploratory abdominal procedures that the doctors ordered. The results always came back negative for a disease, and more than a few medical professionals suggested that I should take an antidepressant because they believed my pain was solely psychological.

Time spent with Mark was a welcome distraction from my medical issues. One day during the summer after my sophomore year, he told me we were going to move a freezer, but I didn't know the freezer was at his sister's home, where I also met his mom and dad. Mary Catherine immediately hugged me and had us all but married; she couldn't stop gushing. She's marvelous, but Mark, in his typical kid-brother fashion, resisted her enthusiasm. He did, however, listen to his dad, who said, "She's a nice heifer. She'll make a good cow. Better marry that one." This was a high compliment from the earthy butcher, and he meant it in the best way.

Mark and I had an argument over nothing on the way home from the meeting with his parents, and that was the end of any serious talk about our becoming a couple, but we remained friends.

As my senior year began, Mark's dad passed away in August 1987, and the grief Mark experienced as a result of his death drew us back together to spend Sunday afternoons sharing a meal at the local Ponderosa Steakhouse week after week.

In January 1988, Mark made the decision to move to Lansdale, Pennsylvania, and attend Calvary Baptist Theological Seminary. Over the winter break, I had been in Idaho where my folks lived at the time, and I was making plans to go to the University of Utah the following fall and pursue a higher degree in nursing. My mom asked about prospective guys, "How about that Mark fella. Didn't you like him?"

"Oh, Mom." I sighed. "I love the guy. But we argue like we're siblings. He's like a brother to me, not a boyfriend."

Well, that "brother o' mine" picked me up at the airport when I flew back to Wisconsin for my last semester, and we attended a symphony in Milwaukee a few days after that. Little did I know at that point his intentions had changed, and he was no longer determined I should marry some young buck, but rather, that I should go ahead and marry the "old" guy who was thirty something and no longer so interested in being single.

Mark asked me to go along to St. Cloud, Wisconsin, to meet some of the rest of his huge family the last weekend in January before he left for seminary. I loved Mark and was very comfortable hanging out with him no matter what we happened to be doing at the time. But I had a menstrual cycle from Hades that weekend! I took pain relievers before we left to meet his sister Jan, her husband, Tom, and their two girls. When we arrived at Jan's, I managed to sit at the dining room table for a little while trying unsuccessfully to carry on a conversation before asking quietly if she had something for the cramping. She gave me a couple of Midol.

This would have been fine, but the cumulative effect of all of the meds caused me to pass out on the way down the stairs. Tom picked me up and carried me to one of his girls' bedrooms. Jan told me she would let Mark know what was wrong, and I bawled and cried out, "No, don't tell him!" She laughed a little and said, "Cori, he has four sisters. He knows about periods."

I wailed, "Yes, but he doesn't need to know I have them!"

What an embarrassing beginning to our more serious relationship; but Mark wasn't put off by my health troubles at that point. Perhaps if he had fully understood the scope of my health issues, he might have run, which was my greatest fear.

I lived in continual anxiety that I would get sick and be considered too much effort to care for and my crying about it all would be reason enough for people to abandon me.

I feared people would leave me because I was altogether too much—too sick, too expensive, too stupid, too little, too weak.

Four weeks and four hours after we said, "I do," I began vomiting from pregnancy hormones. Mark did not understand my inability to keep food down. His sisters and other women he knew were not tossing their cookies at the sight or smell of food; he was at a loss as to why it was such an issue for me.

I also couldn't stand to be kissed, which was very sad since we were newlyweds. I would drive to pick Mark up from work because we had only one vehicle. He would slide into the driver's seat, lean over to kiss me, and I would promptly have to climb out the passenger's side door and puke my guts out in a bush near the parking lot.

One time in particular Mark and I were truly challenged by my physical ailments. In September 1991, on the Friday before my twenty-sixth birthday, I was in a car accident. A semitruck I was driving behind had a load of huge metal pipes that extended beyond the trailer. A few years before, a friend of mine had been beheaded when he ran into a truck with a similar load, so I took note of those dangerous pipes and intentionally kept a safe distance.

It was a God thing.

The truck driver had to come to a sudden stop, and so did I. The woman following me, however, didn't. (I found out later she was tending to a child in the backseat.)

She was going 45 mph and rammed into the tail of my car, shoving me forward and right up to the metal pipes, which almost came through my windshield.

I was taken to the emergency room at Grand View Hospital in Sellersville, Pennsylvania, but it appeared I was fine, just badly shaken.

Monday morning while I was at work, I couldn't speak clearly and the right side of my face was contorted. Paramedics took me from my office at the hospital to the ER. I called Mark and told him I was ill, but I didn't know exactly what was going on. Would he come?

Mark had recently been laid off from Ford Motor Company as a result of the recession combined with the union rules of last hired, first fired. He had a great work ethic, but that wasn't a factor in deciding who kept their jobs at the plant.

He was home caring for our two children when the phone call came. He responded with anger and frustration and asked how he was supposed to get to the hospital when I had the only car in running condition. Being prone to self-sufficiency, he didn't want to ask anyone for help. There is such a thing as compassion fatigue. Add to that Mark's longstanding, visceral, utter dislike of hospitals in general, and the relationship sparks were about to start a forest fire.

I hung up, knowing that my hospital stay was getting on his last nerve. I wasn't sure he was going to come. I lay on the gurney in the ER, tears flowing as I asked God to heal me quickly so Mark would not be unhappy with me or worry about new medical bills challenging our finances, especially while he wasn't employed. I felt so alone and helpless.

Mark did come to the ER but not for a while. A couple hours later he came in with Sarah and Jonathan. They were strapped in the stroller, and I knew immediately Mark had walked the three miles to the hospital. He was fuming.

At that time in our marriage, he saw my physical ailments as a ploy. I had overheard him saying to others, "She has a flair for the dramatic." This cut me to the core. It made my pain, difficulties, and illnesses seem like a cry for attention when, God knows, deep down I wanted to be attended to but not in such a negative, burdensome way.

When Mark came into the ER, he saw that the right side of my face was drooping. The admitting physician and the neurologist didn't know exactly what was going on, but they ordered test after test and were exploring all possibilities, including the big one: brain tumor.

Actually seeing my deformed expression with the right side of my face limp and contorted and hearing the doctors' concerns curbed some of the annoyance Mark had had over the inconvenience of hauling our kiddos to the hospital. Turns out a brain tumor was not the cause of my stroke. It was caused from the car accident I'd had three days before. The whiplash injury I sustained caused a slow leak in my left vertebral artery, which hemorrhaged over the next three days and resulted in the stroke Monday morning.

Mark was unemployed, and now I was, too. Disability covered part of my paycheck for the next nine months while I recovered, and it became an awful yet also wonderful opportunity to trust God in ways we had not had to do previously.

The aneurysm didn't claim my life, but the generalized disruption of my autonomic nervous system has left me with daily challenges. Not a meal goes by when I don't choke. To put it politely, coordinating swallowing efforts with breathing is not something I do well. I have learned to sit at the end of the table so I can make a quick exit if necessary.

The next seventeen years gave us more opportunities to trust God as well as deal with physical health challenges. Crazy enough, in spite of severe health issues, I gave birth to a total of eight children, and our lives continued to move along.

6

THE BROKEN VESSEL

When through fiery trials thy pathway shall lie,
My grace, all-sufficient, shall be thy supply.
The flames shall not hurt thee; I only design
Thy dross to consume and thy gold to refine.

—JOHN KEEN, "HOW FIRM A FOUNDATION,
YE SAINTS OF THE LORD"

In October 2008, when I was forty-three, my health started a steady decline. One morning at 3:00 I stumbled out of bed and headed for the bathroom, hemorrhaging from my uterus and reeling from the intestinal spasms the cramping provoked.

The pain was so severe that I needed Mark's help, but my breath was taken away by the cramping so I couldn't call loudly enough to get his attention. I stood up to go to him and pitched into the corner of the bathroom wall, hitting my head and falling on the floor in a faint. Mark woke up when he heard the loud thud as I fell. He quickly got out of bed and walked to the bathroom. By that time I had managed to stand up again and was propped against the sink, but when he asked me what was wrong, I couldn't answer intelligibly and fainted once again. He caught me before I fell over and carried me to our bed.

I came around again, but because of the lump on my forehead, I lost my memory in the short term, and this confusion on my part scared the man something fierce. He called 911, and I was taken to the hospital and admitted.

The neurologist came to my room a few days later and pulled up a chair next to my bed. I was heavily medicated for the undiagnosed abdominal pain but still recall the conversation and have laughed about it. It was the one light-hearted moment in the midst of such a mess.

"So, tell me what happened," he said.

"I fainted in the bathroom and hit my head when I fell," I explained.

"How did you get up?"

"I guess I tried to walk but fainted again, so Mark carried me to the bedroom."

"He carried you?" the neurologist asked, shaking his head in disbelief.

Not understanding his confusion, I repeated, "Yes, he carried me. I couldn't walk because I kept passing out."

"He picked you up and carried you, seriously? Dead weight?" The doctor was flabbergasted.

"He does this all the time, because it's not unusual for me to black out in the bathroom." I scrunched up my face and narrowed my eyes at him, asking, "Are you saying I'm fat?"

"No, no," he tried to convince himself and me, unsuccessfully. This doctor might not be able to haul his wife around, but my husband has some strong guns. He works out in part because he never knows for sure when he's going to have to haul me up the stairs or out of the bathroom. I had no clue how unusual this talent is in a husband. I've got myself a real keeper!

I was in and out of the operating room for exploratory procedures three times in the next couple of months and was finally admitted in December for a hysterectomy to stop the bleeding. The underlying cause of my physical ailments was yet to be discovered. To recover from all the surgical procedures, I received heavy-duty antibiotics and consumed enough narcotics to knock a 350-pound football player on his rear. This resulted in even more GI spasms.

In January I had a follow-up appointment with Dr. H, the ob-gyn who did the hysterectomy. While waiting to see him, I had to use the restroom, which had muddy puddles on the floor tracked in from other people's boots. Intestinal cramping caused me to have another spell where I grew faint. I detested the idea of landing on the dirty floor, and I managed to stay upright by clinging to the safety bar next to the toilet.

When Dr. H came in to see me, I told him, "I'm so tired of falling on the floor when I have to go to the bathroom." My shoulders were hunched forward; I felt weary and defeated.

He whirled around from the desk where he was getting ready to put my information into the computer. "What? What? You mean the concussion in October wasn't the first time that's happened?" He was shocked.

"Uh no! I've been fainting and falling like this for thirty years," I said. "Isn't that why women go to the bathroom in pairs? If one falls off the pot, the other can call for help?"

I was serious about that inquiry.

My doctor was beyond confused. "Why didn't you say something about this years ago?"

"I did," I protested. "I told the cardiologist when I was working in the ICU I had these spells where my heartbeat flipped out of sync. He told me it's not unusual for people to have transient irregular heartbeats. He looked at me and said I looked pretty good and not to worry about it. I don't want to be whining about every little thing I have that's wrong with me. Shoot! I'd never quit complaining."

What a sweet thing to hear Dr. H say, "I think you've got neurocardiogenic syncope, and you need to get that checked out ASAP."

I was amazed to think there was an actual name for what I was experiencing. I wasn't alone in having fainting problems. The outcome of that conversation resulted in a cardiology appointment where the doctor ordered medications to help with my low blood pressure and heart rate. The medications weren't effective for me, but it was a sincere try.

I fell off the toilet time and again in the next three and a half years. Many episodes resulted in a dreadfully embarrassing and expensive trip to the ER via ambulance. The emergency medical service (EMS) guys would burst into my bathroom and find me in a sweaty, disheveled, half-dressed, disoriented mess. They would then transport me to the hospital again where symptoms could at least be managed.

Food and I had a mostly hateful relationship. Just about everything I ate made me nauseated and caused intestinal spasms. I would come home from work at night, drink a glass of milk, take my meds, and go to bed. I was inadequately nourishing my body, and while I didn't know it at the time, milk is not my friend and actually was doing more harm than good.

I had a colonoscopy around this time, and even though I was heavily sedated to the point of unconsciousness and the pain was supposedly blocked, my gut was so ravaged and inflamed that my body was trying to get off the table. My GI doctor told me he had never seen that happen before.

I was always praying, asking God to fix me. I had a home to run, a family to care for, and a job I loved, but my continuing health issues were royally getting in the way of how I wanted to live my life.

God answered those prayers but not in a way I expected. I found He does not answer prayers, fervent ones, halfway. When I told Him through song and prayers to "take my life and let me be consecrated, Lord, to Thee"—oh boy. The hour before the dawn is the darkest. And the "hour" doesn't mean sixty minutes when it comes to God's perfect timing.

God has also actively controlled the circumstances and people necessary to tumble me head over heels into my worst nightmare where I heard:

"I cannot deal with you."

"I am helpless to do anything for you."

"Why can't you just be okay?"

"Why can't you just do your job?"

"Why are you the way you are?"

"Pull yourself together. You're such a mess."

And I was abandoned by those who were not meant to stay.

I believed my life would never be different. I believed I would always be in pain and, worse yet, falling short of expectations that I not be ill.

Emily and Andrew, my two youngest children, at eight and ten years old respectively, were out to eat with my dad and me one evening. As we sat in the booth waiting for our food, we could see a bunch of teenagers goofing off in the parking lot. One of the guys picked up one of the teen girls to show off his male prowess. He was carrying her in his arms, racing around in circles, while she laughed herself silly and begged him to put her down.

Andrew turned back to the table and asked my dad, "What are they doing?"

My dad said, "Being silly. Guys do that when they're young and dumb. Married men don't carry their wives around like that."

Both of my kids said simultaneously, "My dad does!" And Andrew added, "He carries my mom all the time; only she's not laughing."

Sigh.

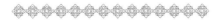

I was sick and tired, really sick and tired, of being sick and tired.

By the fall of 2010, my health grew worse, and my ability to cope exhausted itself.

I felt it would be better not to be here at all than to be continually creating frustration, anger, or disappointment in those I most wanted to please. I was failing miserably. Even more insidious were the doubts that my prayers mattered or that God was listening or cared. It certainly seemed as if He couldn't be bothered with me, and maybe He was even terribly disappointed I had turned out to be such a wreck. I wondered if He thought I was all "wrong" and if in spite of all of the wonderful blessings He had bestowed, He wished I were different and better too.

I am now fully convinced that the silence of God in that hour of need was His blessing in disguise. Hello! I had threatened to check out and somehow quit *life*—not just my job—if He didn't keep His end of the bargain and make my life manageable.

I judged my life as expendable if I couldn't be fixed. I was at the end of my rope and my resources. There appeared to be no hope.

God didn't just allow my trials to linger, but I fully believe He created the perfect storm in December 2010. All the pressure I had been feeling mounted and crashed in with an unprecedented intensity.

At work seven babies under my mantle of care were miscarried or stillborn, and I met with all of their families in my role as a bereavement specialist. Emotionally it was an incredibly taxing week; a typical week had around three or four preterm deaths.

Thursday rolled around, and I got caught on the OB floor with a family whose baby passed away. I needed time and patience to be with them while they grieved and worked through their options for the color of blanket, design on the outfit, and who they wanted to be present for delivery and afterward. In the hours after the baby's death, making decisions was critical to their well-being in the moment *and* for the rest of their lives. Providing ways to make memories helped alleviate some regret and couldn't be accomplished quickly. I was sweating bullets because I was not able to get to the time clock in time to punch out until two hours after my allotted time was up for the week.

I went home that night with a crushed spirit. In spite of my best efforts to scramble and get the job done—and done well—in the given time frame, I had failed.

On Friday I was dreading a call from my boss telling me I had blown it one too many times. I didn't feel as if the hospital directors or the managers who reported to them cared about the reasons I was over my allotted time. All that mattered was the fact that I was. It didn't matter that I had tried.

I was in such despair. My gut was aching and spasming. I couldn't eat and couldn't sleep.

The call from work I was praying for didn't come. I wanted someone to tell me I had been forgiven for the hours I was over or to tell me I had blown it for the last time. I had no resolution on either front. The pressure valve was firmly in place, no leaks allowed.

On Saturday I tried to put one foot in front of the other and attempted to homeschool my younger kids. My nine-year-old sat back in her chair with her arms folded defiantly across her chest and huffed, "I don't know why you're even bothering to try and teach us. It's not like we're learning anything." This was not a new criticism. Good grief, I had been a mother for twenty-one years and endured many a look or comment about my being the world's worst mom. But that day it was the last straw—a light straw to be sure, but the camel's back was already breaking.

Late that afternoon, Mark and I had an argument over an extended family dinner that I did not want to attend. I felt my health issues were considered an undue burden to them, and I had been told I wasn't carrying my end of the load and Mark was doing more than his fair share. A few of his family members had expressed irritation over my weaknesses and the ongoing drama of my being in and out of the hospital.

I didn't just have burdens; I *was* a burden.

Mark didn't know how fragile I felt or how inaccurate I was when evaluating my ability to contribute or be productive. I was *in* pain, and even worse, I believed I *was* a pain.

The certainty that life would never be different loomed over my soul and made me desperate.

On the spur of the moment that evening, I decided to get in the car and drive. I went west. About sixty miles from home I pulled off into a truck stop parking lot.

I sighed as I turned off the engine. I was going to sleep, and I was going to wake up in heaven.

I reached in my purse and found the bottle of Ambien. I fiddled with the cap and spilled out a handful. Just before I swallowed them, I wept, and the little girl inside of me said, *Jesus, please don't be mad at me.*

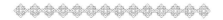

God was not done with me yet even if I had decided I was.

I woke up several hours after I had swallowed about thirty of the sleeping pills. The front of my coat, in addition to the car seat and door, was covered in vomit. I didn't slip away and go to heaven in my sleep. Instead, I had only made things worse.

I was still too drugged to drive but not fully conscious enough to realize it. Only God knows how I did it, my fingers fumbling about, but I managed to completely wipe everything out on my phone except for my home phone number. I called Mark and managed to tell him what I had done, but I couldn't process what he was telling me.

I drove down the road while talking on the cell phone. My vision was impaired to the extent that all was blackness when I tried to focus my eyes on the road ahead. But I had a little peripheral vision and was able to see a road sign off the passenger's side of the car. I told Mark what the sign said.

Somehow I "drove" through the busy city of Fond du

Lac, four-lane highways, numerous stoplights, and miles of dark country road before what Mark was saying registered. He wasn't angry, but rather he was coming with Joshua and Tamara, my future daughter-in-law, to find me, and he would drive my car the rest of the way. It finally sunk in he was pleading with me to please, pull over!

I had been advised in college by a fellow student, "If you're going to try and commit suicide, don't do it in your own hometown. You'll never live it down if you fail."

This sounded like sage advice at the time, and I tucked it away, cringing now with how foolish it is in truth. That's one of the lame reasons I drove an hour down the road before pulling off. As it ended up, my husband found me parked on the side of a road and took me to the emergency room at the very hospital I worked at. The warning from my college days rang in my head when I awakened enough to realize where I was.

My decision to go to sleep and wake up in heaven had not been well thought out. The ER doctor asked me what I thought I was doing. He said, "You're a nurse. You should know sleeping pills don't work. Your body throws up what you don't need. Seriously?"

I shrugged my shoulders in defeat and shook my head in weariness, closing my eyes to shut everyone out. I despaired that not only had I failed to live effectively, but I also couldn't even die properly, and I was now facing all the backlash from my stupidity.

I was admitted to our local psych ward at a different facility on Sunday afternoon under the state's chapter 51 statute.

The psychiatrist who met with Mark and me told us, "You gotta figure out what's up here and what's going to be different moving forward. This wasn't a serious attempt to end your life, but something's gotta change."

After spending several hours with me, Mark went home to be with our kids. I wasn't allowed to go home but was encouraged to spend time in the day room and watch the Packers football game that evening with the other patients on the unit. I looked around, and my first thought was *I'm not one of you people. I don't need to be here.* Shame immediately engulfed me. Who did I think I was to say they were "you people" and I wasn't one of them? They were hurting just as I was, maybe for different reasons, but hurting just the same.

The next morning Mark came in early and the doctor showed up at 7:00 to meet with Mark and me.

I told him, "You know, my health is lousy, and my job is incredibly stressful; I have a lot on my plate, but nobody is holding a gun to my head saying I have to do any of this. Something must change, and I don't know what that will be, but I will not be pressed on all sides and made to feel this desperate and without options again."

He told both of us that he truly didn't think it was a chapter 51 case, and so he was dismissing it. Discharge orders were in by 7:30 a.m. I went home to reevaluate and get my life together.

My husband was okay with me quitting my job if that's what I wanted, but he wisely didn't force a decision either way. I lay on the floor of my bedroom, facedown, weeping, in as humble a posture as I could manage, and prayed: "God, I cannot believe I have to get up and walk out of this room and go back to work. I cannot hide in my home for the rest of my days and avoid people forever. I have no idea how I am going to do this, but You decided it was not ending this way, so show up for me. I need You to carry me now. I haven't the strength to do it alone."

The fallout from my actions spread farther than I had bargained.

Most people shouldn't have had any clue what happened, but word gets around in a small town, and there was no hiding it. I was the most surprised at the backlash of anger, the complete lack of compassion on the part of some friends, family, and acquaintances. One coworker narrowed her eyes and through clenched teeth said, "You call your bereavement program Hope After Loss Organization. What right do you have to tell anyone about hope after anything?"

But my hope wasn't in me. Psalm 107 was there for people who had been foolish. They cried out to the Lord in their distress, and He delivered them. He didn't react to their heartfelt cry for redemption with scorn, saying, "You blew it, you idiot. Fix it yourself." No, He had compassion and offered forgiveness and restoration.

I can wish I had a spotless record, but I do not.

Instead of wasting time wishing away the past or that it was different or that I was a better person, I have taken to heart some wise advice from Dr. John Piper:

> "You believe with all your might in justification
> by grace alone through faith alone on the basis of
> Christ's righteousness alone to the glory of God
> alone. And when you stumble and act inconsis-
> tently with that profession of glorious acceptance,
> you hate it. You get up. You confess your sins and

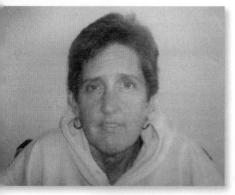

LEFT: Intake photo at Sanoviv Medical Institute. So sick and weak I was unable to stand long enough to shower.

RIGHT: Mary Elisbeth, Johanna, Emmalynn, Charity, and myself at the Wynonna Judd concert.

BELOW: Trying to memorize the feel of the weight of her little body in my arms, knowing she wouldn't be in them for very long.

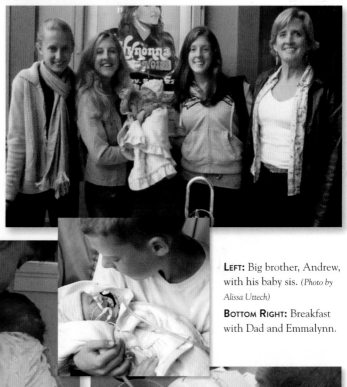

LEFT: Big brother, Andrew, with his baby sis. *(Photo by Alissa Uttech)*

BOTTOM RIGHT: Breakfast with Dad and Emmalynn.

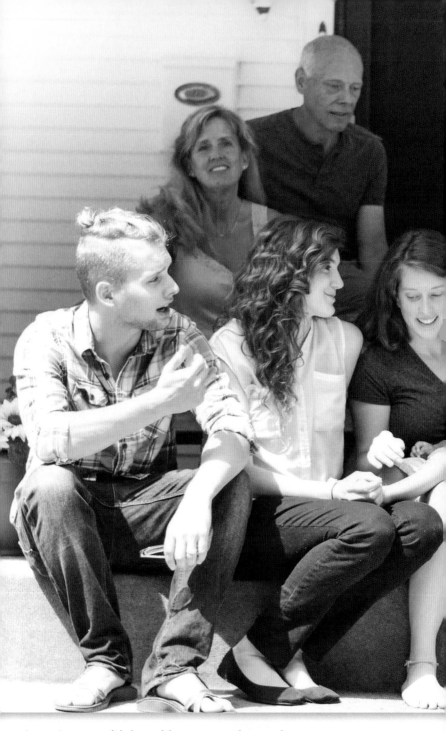

ABOVE: A more candid photo of the gang on our front porch.

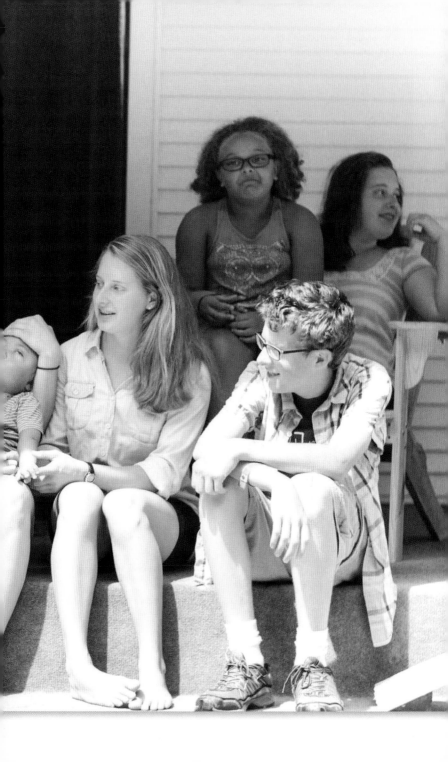

ALL: Stephanie Smith from Lenses for Love caught a little of the love our Charlie receives from Mom and Dad and the older siblings.

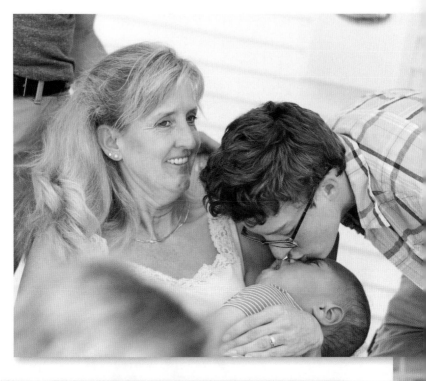

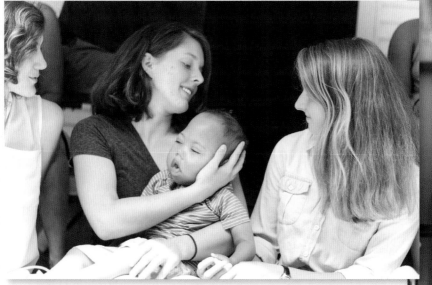

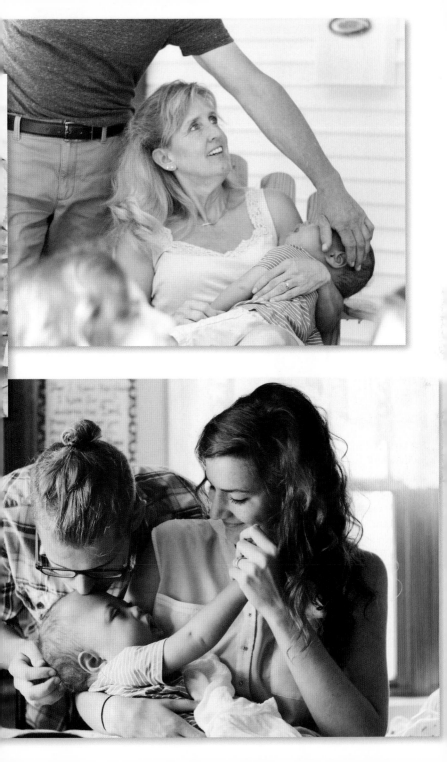

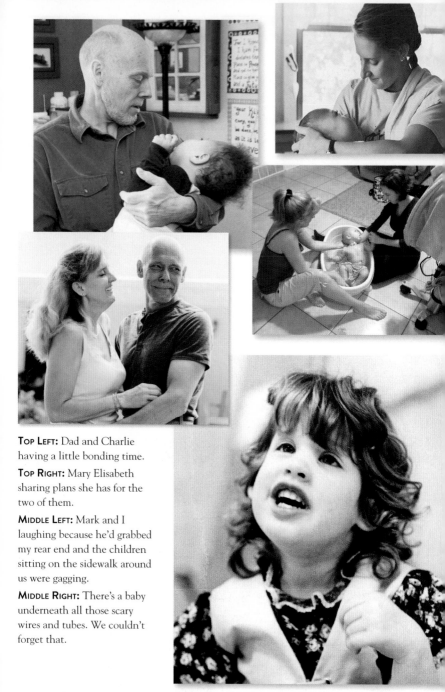

TOP LEFT: Dad and Charlie having a little bonding time.

TOP RIGHT: Mary Elisabeth sharing plans she has for the two of them.

MIDDLE LEFT: Mark and I laughing because he'd grabbed my rear end and the children sitting on the sidewalk around us were gagging.

MIDDLE RIGHT: There's a baby underneath all those scary wires and tubes. We couldn't forget that.

ABOVE: My sister, Amie, at about three years old, the time wh[en] she liked to play with the door and spring and giggle herself silly.

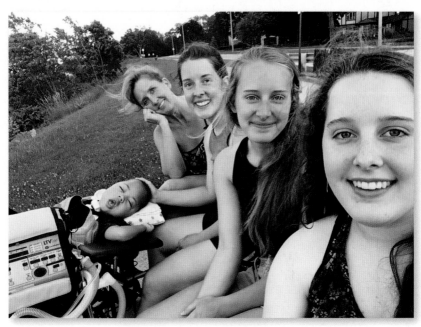

ABOVE: A quick walk along Lake Michigan with the sisters and little bro.

BELOW: Hail, hail, some of the gang is here!

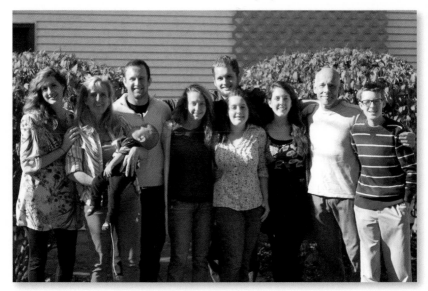

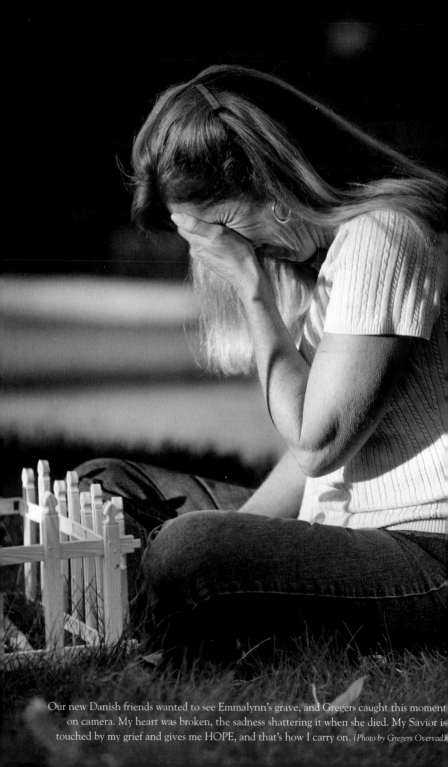

Our new Danish friends wanted to see Emmalynn's grave, and Gregers caught this moment on camera. My heart was broken, the sadness shattering it when she died. My Savior is touched by my grief and gives me HOPE, and that's how I carry on. *(Photo by Gregers Overvad)*

you keep on going, because his righteous is the bottom line, not yours. His righteousness is the bottom line."[1]

My hope was in God, but I had no short, pat answer for my coworker, so I shrugged my shoulders and once more threw myself at Jesus' chest and asked for mercy and grace.

I'm quite aware that there are those who still feel my life is a joke and that I haven't lived up to what I have "preached" to be true. This is a source of grief that I brought shame to Jesus' name even though it was my decision, not His, to be a fool.

One valuable lesson learned from the whole experience is that no challenge I have—whether it be a job, a relationship, or my inability to control my health—is worth taking my own life. I can choose not to be defined by the roles I play in my life: a mom, a wife, a friend, an employee. I can choose to be strong should those roles change or be taken away from me. What I do does not define who I am. Nothing should have that kind of power over my heart and mind and soul.

My desire to be a "rock star" and make people happy was an elusive pursuit and a futile one. Living for the approval of others isn't safe. How many folks need to think I'm good or amazing or worthwhile? There will always be somebody who is unhappy with me.

If life's about being good enough, I'm utterly overdrawn at the bank.

What a precious gift God gave me to help me fall completely short and not be enough. This concept is spelled out in Romans 3:23: "All have sinned and fall short of the glory of God" (NIV).

This verse is for everyone. No one is good. No one is enough. We're all sinners. Trying to keep our lives together and be as good as possible doesn't work.

How freeing to *finally* quit trying so hard to be good enough. It's all because of Jesus that I'm alive and have anything good going on in my life.

The enemy taunted me for years, pointing out my flaws! The subtlety by which he accuses is this: he uses portions of the truth—I am all those things I never wanted to be.

And now when the enemy tosses my miserable and multiple failures in my face, I imagine seeing Jesus walking along the Sea of Galilee. He looks up and sees me. His face breaks into a huge grin, and He beckons me with His whole arm, not just a couple of fingers, to come to Him, to come running. He tosses both arms wide and envelops me in a hug and draws me close to His side. He says, *I love you. I died, lady. I died for you. For all your sins. For all your mess. You are not too much for Me. Come, walk with Me here; tell Me about your day. I'm listening, and I am not wishing you were different or better. You are loved with an everlasting love. You. Are. Mine.*

And then the accuser, the enemy of my soul, slips away, defeated in the moment, and ultimately will be defeated forever.

Let me be clear, I also feel as though I got a good hard spanking from my heavenly Father. He could have allowed me to die, but He did not. He was not done with me yet, and my life was not going to end at a truck stop. The grace He lavished on me and on my family was crazy amazing. He scared me straight, and it takes my breath away when I contemplate all the ways He protected me when I would not and could not protect myself. God preserved me through terrible hardship in the pursuit of true health and not simply a masked semblance of it. Even with all I continued to endure in the next eighteen months, I was not suicidal. It's not my decision to dictate to Him how and when I'm going to die. He is the Father, and I am the child. He is in charge of that business, and it's not mine to meddle with.

In the article "Lay Aside the Weight of Perfection," author Jon Bloom summarizes why I believe God didn't simply *allow* struggles in my life but actually *caused* them. God was not against me and wanting to expose all my faults maliciously; rather, He did it out of love so I would quit striving for something I would never be able to attain.

> "God is calling us to the wonderfully refreshing experience of getting our eyes off ourselves and how we're measuring up, and onto Jesus (Hebrews 12:2). He wants us to stop pursuing or being paralyzed by perfectionism so we are free to pursue love (1 Corinthians 14:1; 1 Timothy 1:5) and pursue trusting him with all our hearts (Proverbs 3:5). And if perfectionism has an inordinate influence on us, God will mercifully design circumstances to defeat our best efforts to fight sin "successfully" until we learn where our freedom really comes from.
>
> In Christ, you are free! You are free to follow Jesus imperfectly. You are free to fight the fight of faith defectively, because that's the only way you will ever fight for faith in this age."[2]

For years Satan had victory over my emotional and mental health because of severe physical illnesses. His goal was to devour me and to leave me faithless. With a sob catching in my throat and a heavy, settled surety of heart, I can now declare, "My God is good." Period. No catches, no conditions, no quid pro quo. However, I couldn't declare those truths fully without first experiencing a depth of suffering I couldn't fathom enduring or surviving.

Establishing His authority over the timing of my death was essential because I couldn't have endured the coming storm without it.

7

THE DARK BEFORE
THE DAWN

When through the deep waters I call thee to go,
The rivers of sorrow shall not overflow;
For I will be with thee thy troubles to bless
And sanctify to thee thy deepest distress.

—JOHN KEEN, "HOW FIRM A FOUNDATION,
YE SAINTS OF THE LORD"

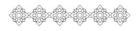

In July 2011 I had been given a new journal by one of the moms I worked with while a bereavement specialist with HALO. The journal had the "Footprints" poem motif illustrated on the cover, the familiar single set of footprints in the sand. There is only one entry:

> *Dear God, The psalm that says You brought me up out of a horrible pit and set my feet on a rock. . . . I cringe at being in the pit. I find myself afraid of what fires You've got to take me through to purify my inner woman. I don't want to be afraid. Perfect love casts out fear. Your love is perfect; mine is not. I want to trust You more than I want to avoid the pain that comes with growth.*
>
> *Help me.*

As the summer unfolded, I had no idea that God was going to answer my heartfelt prayers by plunging me into a horribly terrifying pit.

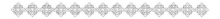

Over the years, doctors had prescribed a number of different medications to help me deal with the symptoms of my then undiagnosed autoimmune diseases. For years I had been in and out of the hospital seeking a diagnosis for my abdominal pain. My gut feeling—pun intended—is that when doctors don't know for sure why someone has abdominal pain, the diagnosis is irritable bowel syndrome (IBS). Those three little letters are one giant garbage can of festering symptoms: spasms, constipation, diarrhea, excessive gas, indigestion, and vomiting.

In late July 2011, I attended the Rachel's Vineyard Leadership Conference in Pennsylvania since the arrangements had already been made for me to go and learn more about grief counseling to enhance my work as a bereavement specialist with HALO.

At the conference I asked a dear friend to pray with me and for me. We knelt beside her bed, and I poured out my heart, asking God for direction. Financially, I couldn't just walk away from my job, but my health was failing and I couldn't keep up with the demands at both work and home. I was bewildered and begging God for wisdom because I didn't have a clue how He was going to sort out the tangled threads of my life.

Throughout the conference, all was not well in my abdominal world, but I didn't understand the severity of what was happening until I returned home. A couple of days later, I was in so much pain at work I notified my boss and went to the ER because I feared I would faint and end up with another concussion related to the syncope.

The ER doctor examined me and said I had a deep anal fissure. (Please forgive me if revealing this is too much information. I do know some of you may be squeamish, but this is the way it happened.) The intense pain was causing my heart to go into syncope. He gave me an injection of lidocaine to mask the pain, and I was released.

My world turned upside down after that. The fissure would not heal. The pain was excruciating, and I couldn't find relief even with strong narcotics accompanied by meds to control the vomiting. I was in and out of the ER for days afterward. Finally, I was referred to a specialist in Green Bay.

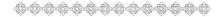

After a barium bowel study, in addition to the fissure, the doctor pointed out the presence of four issues that were much more serious—a sigmoidocele, a rectocele, an enterocoele, and a cystocele. Basically my lower intestinal organs were either dropping, collapsing, and/or bulging in the wrong places.

The specialist told us that while the fissure was the most painful, it was the least of my problems. Everything in my pelvis was sitting in a heap, in part due to having eight pregnancies, hormone changes, IBS, and the hysterectomy in 2008. I was at huge risk of a complete bowel obstruction. I pictured a train wreck with a number of cars piled every which way on top of one another and none of them on the track where they were supposed to be.

Even though the news was bad, a part of me was satisfied that at least I was getting some answers. But what the doctor said next felt like a slap in the face: he declared himself too old to deal with a case this extreme. He wouldn't take me on as a patient.

At this point I had no idea where to find treatment. Three of my girlfriends did some research and thought the Mayo Clinic might offer a solution. They dropped everything they had going on in order to drive six hours to Rochester. We arrived about midnight, barely making it to the ER, and I spent four hours getting IV medications, which temporarily relieved the excruciating pain. My friends got Charity and me settled in a hotel across the street from the hospital, paying for the room, and then drove all the way home. Because I was in terrible pain night after night, Charity would put me in a wheelchair and roll me to the ER. And night after night I would beg someone, *anyone* to please fix me.

My body was my enemy, and I had no way to eliminate the pain or escape from it. After seeing a number of doctors and having a radiologist review the barium study from Green Bay, he erroneously determined I had no bowel issues.

On the tenth morning, a surgeon did a minor procedure to help the pain from the fissure and released me from care. Mark and Mary Elisabeth drove to pick up Charity and me to go home. The injected anesthetic carried me through the six-hour drive, but I was home only hours when the pain came back again in waves.

My husband was desperate and called my ob-gyn, Dr. H, who knew me and knew that if I said I was in pain, I was. He advised that we go to the ER at our local hospital and he would make sure I was admitted. Mark brought me there, and I was given a consultation with our local surgeon. He was able to relieve the pressure on the fissure so I could finally begin healing there. He told me he was not skilled enough to surgically fix the collapse of my lower internal organs.

The next referral took me to Milwaukee to no avail because the doctor wouldn't even examine me, and then to Rush University Medical Center in Chicago. There was no help to be found there for me either.

The despair, frustration, and confusion I felt were downright palpable. How could I be making this stuff up? The Green Bay specialist said my GI problems were so bad he wouldn't treat me. My local surgeon said my problem was too difficult for him to fix. So how could the doctors at Mayo and at Rush both say my issues didn't even exist? How could I be too much trouble to several physicians but other doctors couldn't even say that I had a problem?

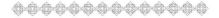

In November, after having spent ten days chasing appointments in Chicago, I was referred to doctors in West Allis, Wisconsin, who weren't afraid to see me or do surgery for me.

After meeting with these two doctors in West Allis, the GI surgeon examined me and looked at my previous test results. "Oh yeah," she said, "you're a mess." I gave a sigh of relief. At least she knew it wasn't all in my mind!

By now it was late November, and my surgery could not be scheduled until mid-January. Despite my poor health, I still had long, full, beautiful hair, and one day in December 2011, I leaned against the sink and arranged my hair in six sections. Then I began to cut off the ponytails to give to Locks of Love.

It was a desperate move. I did it in part because I did not have the strength to stand up in the shower, but more than that, it was an utter humbling before God. If having long and beautiful hair was in any way vain, then the cause for my vanity was now gone. Mark walked in while I was on ponytail number three. When he saw what I was doing, his eyes welled up with tears. His chest heaved with sobs as he turned and left the bathroom, visibly helpless to do anything for me or to change the situation for the better. After the ponytails were cut, I weakly took his hair clippers to my head and shaved off the rest of it.

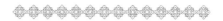

When January 2012 rolled around and it was time for my surgery, my requests for interventions to help me deal with the procedures and pain were ignored or unable to be accomplished. I'm not going to go into medical detail, but suffice it to say, after surgery to remove fourteen inches of my colon and correct some of the other more life-threatening issues, nothing in my lower abdomen was in a natural position anymore,* resulting in permanent damage that cannot be remedied.

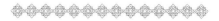

Going back and reliving the pain and the disappointment I felt after the surgery is extremely difficult. My expectations of how I thought things should be and how my health problems and pain should be managed were not met. It wasn't that most of the doctors I saw weren't wonderful, kind people, but they simply couldn't do anything more medically than they were doing.

* rectopexy

I was discharged from the hospital mid-January, but the spasming in my colon did not go away, and I had new troubles because of scar tissue buildup. Mark and I went to see the GI surgeon in March. I told her I was in considerable pain because adhesions had formed that were affecting my bladder. She had done her best to do a very low incision to remove my sigmoid in order not to have adhesions form, which would constrict my small bowel. Thank God for that, but the pain when my bladder was full or emptying was nauseating, and nothing could be done because opening me up again would just cause more scar tissue to form, a no-win situation.

As we sat there with her and I explained the confusion over my painful GI symptoms still remaining, she pushed her stool back into the corner, crossed her legs, sighed, and said, "There's a new study out that says people with IBS have normal peristalsis [bowel contractions], they just perceive it as pain, but it really isn't painful. You're obviously struggling and depressed. Maybe you need to see a psychiatrist and get some help for it." She stood then, shrugged her shoulders slightly, looked at me with pity, and excused herself.

I didn't think I could be knocked down any further. Yeah, I could consider being depressed part of my issues, understandably so, but her words intimating the debilitating pain was a figment of my imagination made me feel as if I had been swallowed up in a dark hole.

My dear husband shook his head in disbelief and muttered, "Right. It's not painful, just normal peristalsis that wakes you up out of a sound sleep at 2:00 a.m. and causes you to stagger to the bathroom and pass out. I don't think so. Let's get out of here."

I spent most of my time in bed in the fetal position. The fear of being left with no recourse or hope made me resort to anger in defense. I had no filter on my mouth anymore. The drugs and the pain left me saying whatever I wanted to whomever was in my path, but Mark received the worst of it.

He has told me it was the most frightening to him when I would not respond at all. He would purposely goad me to get a reaction because even an angry response showed I still had some spark. I have been told numerous times that the fact he didn't hightail it out of the marriage is extraordinary. Mark did not stay because it was fun. He did not stay because I was meeting his needs. He didn't even stay because he had any feelings of warm, fuzzy love. The reason the man did not abandon me is because God enabled him to put his head down, "grab the bull by the horns," and carry on. Mark had vowed "I do," in sickness and in health and for richer and poorer. What we both hoped for on our wedding day was continued health and some riches. Our marriage would not have survived had God not used my husband's steadfast determination not to quit to sustain him day after day in such bleak, unrelenting circumstances.

I'm sure Mark cried a number of times during my extended illness, but he usually did not cry in front of me. One day he did tell me—but only once—"We're going to get through this."

Wanting him to feel the depth of my pain too, I looked at him and, practically hissing, said, "*We* are not in pain. *I* am in pain. You have no idea what I'm going through. *We* are not going to get through anything!"

At one point I got hysterical and shouted, "I hate you! I hate you!"

He bowed his head, and barely glancing back up, he said softly, "You can't say that to me. I know you're in pain, but I'm trying. You just can't say that to me." He walked away with his shoulders slumped in defeat.

Oh how I wanted to escape, out of my house, out of my family, out of my pain, and I had nowhere to go. I couldn't function physically. I couldn't drive. Mark had hidden the car keys so I wouldn't be able to attempt to do so either. Okay, so I could stumble to the bathroom a couple of times a day, but that was it. The helplessness and the pain wore me to a frazzle.

At one point I decided to run away. I don't know how I did it, but I walked to the bus station in downtown Sheboygan, about a mile and a half from my house. I had my purse and some money I had taken out of our savings account. I was too weak to carry a suitcase. I wanted to get on a bus and maybe go to Florida where it was warm and I could lie on the beach and soak up the sun, possibly relieving some of the pain I was in.

I was under the influence of the Valium and narcotics prescribed for my pain, so I was not able to think as clearly as the situation called for. I couldn't quite make out the bus schedule, but the man who oversaw the station informed me there wouldn't be another bus to Chicago until evening. It was only 11:00 a.m. I was getting hungry and feeling faint. How in the world was I going to survive if I left? I could picture a couple of dear people I loved finding me on their doorstep and the fear and uneasiness their eyes would reflect upon seeing me in my unstable state. They might have cared about me a lot, but they wouldn't want me. I was too much to handle, and even the bravest souls in my life would quail and were not up for the task of helping me.

The sobering realization came over me. I had no place to go. I couldn't get out of the pain I was in, and nobody else wanted me to be with them because they were helpless to do anything for me. My family may have not been able to redeem my life from the pit I was in, but they were the only ones who were willing to stay by me day after incredibly long, painful day. I made my way home again and have no recollection of getting there.

Mark heroically and tenaciously clung to the hope that God had not abandoned us, and even that grated on my nerves because I could not see where having faith in God was helpful. God had the power to relieve this suffering with a word, but He didn't. Why in the world was His silence so deafening?

I didn't save my caustic words just for family. A long-time friend, Darin, who was in treatment for kidney failure, came and sat by my bedside day after day. He would talk about everything and nothing and demand that I get out of bed and walk down the hallway. I would wearily turn my face toward him and pathetically say, "Can you not see I'm in no shape to move out of this bed. I cannot breathe without pain, let alone move my body without it hurting. Go! Away!"

He would continue to sit in the rocking chair and tell me, "I'm not leaving until you walk down the hall. You can walk twenty feet, then get back into bed."

"And what about *no* can you not understand?" I would say. "Leave me alone!"

"I will, as soon as you get out of that bed and walk."

"If you don't get out of my room, I am going to hurt you!"

"Fine. But you will have to get out of bed in order to

come over here and hurt me, so let's be doing it."

I could have fallen back asleep and tolerated his presence, but he wouldn't give up. He kept talking and talking about nothing intelligent or pertinent to my life, and I finally pushed back the covers. Wincing in pain and cussing at him all the while, I sat up, eased out of bed, walked down the hall and back again, then climbed back into bed and rolled toward the wall away from him.

"Nice going!" he would cheerfully quip. "I'll be back tomorrow."

"Don't let the door hit you in the butt on the way out," was my pleasant, heartfelt response to his promise not to leave me alone.

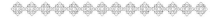

A plaque hangs on my bedroom wall that my son Jonathan gave me for Christmas in 2010. It's a picture of a completely barren tree in a field covered with snow. A single set of footprints can be seen in the snow. And like my journal, the line from the "Footprints" poem—"When you see only one set of footprints, it was then that I carried you"—is written in script across the gray landscape, totally devoid of color. I looked at that plaque regularly and at one point asked Jesus in utter defeat, tears flowing, "Why do I have to be carried? I'd much rather be able to carry my own weight and walk."

By April 2012, I was completely bedridden, getting up only to use the bathroom. Nearly everything I ate caused me intestinal distress, and I hardly swallowed anything. I moaned in pain whenever I adjusted my position in bed, whether awake or asleep. There was nothing any of the doctors I had seen could do. They were baffled at my physical decline. I was stuck. I soaked my pillow with tears, asking in confusion why I was still living, if you could call my existence living. How could this be bringing any glory to God?

All the prayers offered appeared useless. What was the point of praying when day in and day out I was still lying in that bed? Mark had to homeschool the kids and chauffeur them to appointments without my help. My teen girls came alongside Mark and took on the housework—the vacuuming and mopping, the dozen loads of laundry per week, the endless cycle of cooking and dishwashing. At times they felt irritated and ornery, even bitter about having to help clean or make meals. Those were normally my jobs, and I was failing miserably at them. So to say my children had an undercurrent of tension and rebellion in their hearts would be a colossal understatement.

There was no larking about with a song in our hearts. Our family was in mourning. We were surviving. With no end in sight. I was too sick to live and not sick enough to die. Life faded to gray and we had little hope color would ever enter into it again.

My son Andrew was twelve years old at the time and was struggling at school. He lived in constant fear of coming home and learning that I had been admitted to the hospital again or having to call 911 and watch the EMTs haul me out or coming home to find out I had died.

God's ways are not our ways, and His thoughts are not our thoughts (Isaiah 55:8–9). My children also needed to have their faith shaken to the core. Any false assumptions about the goodness of God corresponding to the goodness of our circumstances needed to be sifted.

We praise God for being good because our mortgage is paid, our children are healthy, or the new job came through. We give thanks for favorable things and circumstances. But what happens when all our prayers appear to go unheard and our circumstances are *not* favorable? Does God become evil then? Is His character so fickle that when my life is good, He is good, and when it's not, somehow He has changed?

I'm an avid reader, but because of the medications I was taking for the pain and spasming, I couldn't focus enough to read more than a few sentences at a time. A couple of our dearest friends, Todd and Kelly, called me one afternoon. I asked them in desperation, "Why is God not taking me home? Why is He leaving me to barely exist, wanting to die but not able to do so?" There was silence on the other end of the phone, but then they quietly said to me, "We don't know. We don't know, Cori." They could not fix it for me, and that fact had made most people disappear. But then Todd offered gently, "I have found comfort in listening to Dr. John Piper's sermons on *Suffering and the Sovereignty of God.* I'll send you the website link, and maybe it will be a way for you to make some sense of this."

I looked up desiringgod.org as Todd had suggested. Day after day, night after night when I could not sleep because I was hurting so badly from my entire body being in a state of inflammation, I would listen to Dr. Piper's messages. I played his series about Job over and over and over again. I would fall asleep listening to the words he was speaking, and God literally used them to help clear my thinking in spite of the drugs I was taking. I did not lose my mind in complete despair over the suffering I was enduring.

Later that month a friend of ours at church waded into our suffering and gave us a brochure about Sanoviv Medical Institute in Rosarito, Mexico. The brochure featured a spa-like resort, complete with saltwater swimming pools and an ocean view. I laughed when I saw it, much like Sarah did when told she was going to have a baby at ninety. Yeah, right. Not.

We lacked the $15,000 in up-front money needed to secure a spot. This was a sure sign to me that it was a stupid idea and not worth taking a second look. Mark, however, researched the institute thoroughly and was convinced it was the answer to all the tears and prayers he had cried and prayed.

Another friend, Mike, came over and handed us a check for $15,000. His motive wasn't completely altruistic. He told us with a wink, "I don't want your kids. I don't need eight kids hanging out at my farm. If you die, I'm gonna get 'em, and I don't need that kind of hassle in my life. Get yourself to that hospital in Mexico."

I didn't want to go.

Mark badgered me day after day, telling me I had no choice. He was not paying for a funeral before we exhausted this possibility.

He did not care that I did not want to go.

He did not care that I did not care.

Mark is a rock and can be even more stubborn and mule-headed than I. As proof of this, he put me on a plane. Mark didn't have a passport, so he couldn't go with me. He needed to stay home and take care of the kids. I had to go alone 95 percent against my will.

I have little recollection of my trip to Mexico. I know we had to be up at 3:00 a.m., and my husband drove me to the airport and put me in a wheelchair. The man in charge took me through security to the plane, where I moved into my seat. I was in so much pain I could hardly breathe, and my medications were barely making it tolerable. My fervent prayer was that I would not be sick and unable to get to the bathroom in time or that I would not be stuck in the restroom while others grew impatient waiting for me to exit.

I was transported from the plane to the baggage claim area and picked up by one of the many kind people who work for Sanoviv. I lay down in the seat of the van and dozed fitfully until we arrived at the hospital. My doctors at Sanoviv had their work cut out for them, in part because I was so discouraged about the decline of my physical health. I was not feeling up to the challenge or able to engage in my own healing. I was too weak to try or to care.

The staff at Sanoviv gave back my life to me in many more ways than just the physical realm. I felt as if I had to go through the even darker shadows of death before I found healing. I had deep-seated fears over being more trouble than I was worth and that I would be abandoned as a result. Add to that the crushing disappointment over multiple medications, treatments, surgeries, and procedures that were not helping. The root causes of my autoimmune diseases had yet to be addressed so true healing could take place. Mere symptom control was not cutting it anymore, no way, no how.

Several days after being admitted, the detoxification from all the drugs I had been taking as well as the physical demise I had endured got the best of me. I felt more hopeless and helpless than ever before. The drug withdrawal caused me to have nightmares, and there was no help for that. I called my husband on Friday, sobbing and resigned to the fact that I could not be helped. The physical pain was unbearable.

Dr. Francisco, the primary doctor in charge of evaluating my treatments looked at me one day with tenderness and compassion and said quietly but with intensity, "I believe I can help you. I know you do not believe right now, but I will believe for the both of us."

A little while later, one of the housekeepers entered my room. In her limited English, she asked and motioned with her hands if she could pray for me. I nodded yes, and even that hurt as my head was splitting with pain. She laid a tiny, cool hand on my forehead and proceeded to pray with deep, intense fervency. I understood only the name *Jesucristo*, which she murmured repeatedly. When finished, she gently kissed the area where she had placed her hand on my head and then left as soundlessly as she had come in.

The strange thing was, she wasn't even the housekeeper assigned to my room but apparently had felt compelled to come pray for me. I did not speak to or see her again the rest of my stay.

The oppressive agony I was experiencing did not immediately lift, but that night my dreams were not quite as terrifying. I awoke on Sunday morning with less pain than I'd had in more than a year. I felt a spark of hope, but by no means was it even a candle flame. I guardedly thought, *Okay, maybe it's going to be all right, or at least better than I'd thought.* Sanoviv's medical approach is to decrease or eliminate inflammation at the cellular level and provide health nutritionally and medically with supplements and treatments. The underlying philosophy is that if the body has what it needs to function and toxic substances—certain food, drugs, and environmental pollutants—are eliminated, it can heal.

Everything at Sanoviv is given great thought, from

the food, to the water, to the clothing and bedding, to the aesthetically pleasant surroundings and the medical treatments for diseases.

I had no idea how necessary it was to have such a beautifully serene place to endure the medical treatments prescribed, and those pools, one of them quite warm, were the only way my muscles would stop cramping and aching. Unable to sleep because of the pain, I would go down to them at 1:00 a.m. and slip in for an hour to relax enough to be able to sleep.

I spent most of my mornings waking up and crying for thirty minutes, praying for God to help me get out of bed. I would then make myself go to the nurses' station and receive the prescribed injections, the IVs, or whatever else was on my program. A battle was going on for my life. It was not easy, light warfare. I had told God for years that I wasn't a soldier. But I was required to be tougher than I had ever needed to be in my life, and He was there to strengthen and enable me to do what was required. A warrior emerged in those mornings when I battled with my desires to shrink back from the painful procedures and treatments. I instead gathered my wits and waded into the pain designed to heal.

I was humanly alone for the most part in having to deal with the process. I was isolated, and God met me in that place in ways I could not have anticipated. I know firsthand what it's like to be at your wit's end with no solutions offered except misery and death. I can also say with deep assurance, "Yea, though I walk through the valley of the shadow of death, I will fear no evil; for You are with me; Your rod and Your staff, they comfort me" (Psalm 23:4 NKJV).

My health has been restored in a great measure on all

fronts. I still have a number of autoimmune diseases, but according to the Sanoviv mind-set, I don't mess around trying to medicate the individual symptoms; instead, I continue to carefully control my diet and my coping mechanisms for the stress in my life to keep my inflammation levels a pile of coals rather than the active, raging fire they have been. I will not be cured this side of heaven, but I have been given a new lease on life and am able to live remarkably well now compared to the difficulties I faced for decades.

God carried me through the valleys. He preserved me through my attempts to alienate all who loved and cared for me. Those He wanted to stay did so. I was not ever truly abandoned, and this fear I cowered under for years had the power shaken out of it, and fear of abandonment does not hold sway over my life anymore!

One of my heroes is Joni Eareckson Tada. She has thanked God from a deep place in her heart for all she has endured as a quadriplegic. This act is humanly flabbergasting, and the only way she can genuinely do it is because Jesus has supernaturally given her a heart of joy. She wrote the following in regard to her own sufferings:

> "And I get to become like Him in this life. I get to experience the intimate fellowship of sharing in His sufferings, the sweetness and the preciousness of the Savior. I become holy as He is holy. O God, "you will make me full of gladness with your presence" (Acts 2:28 ESV)."[1]

The song lyrics from "Amazing Grace"—"I once was lost and now am found"—also summarize my experience.

Those words would not have the gravity and glory they deserve if my plight had been only a slight detour. I was at a complete dead end before God lifted me out of the pit. I endured a hurricane, not a spring shower. I have my feet on the Rock of Ages, and He has sheltered me in the midst of the storms.

8

THE TIGHT FIST OF FEAR

Fear not, I am with thee, oh, be not dismayed,
For I am thy God and will still give thee aid;
I'll strengthen thee, help thee, and cause thee to stand,
Upheld by My righteous, omnipotent hand.

—JOHN KEEN, "HOW FIRM A FOUNDATION,
YE SAINTS OF THE LORD"

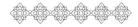

When I was sixteen and a sophomore in high school, my dad took me to get my driver's license. At the time I thought it was because I was nearly an adult and mature for my age; now I know it had more to do with his being sick and tired of running my brothers and me back and forth to school and sports activities. After I got my license and what I assumed was newfound freedom, I felt as if I had my dad's blessing to go wherever I liked. A couple of weeks later I discovered a library. I found a whole row of "racy" novels by Grace Livingston Hill. I sat down on a couch and read one of them in an hour. *Honor Girl* was something akin to *Seven Brides for Seven Brothers* where Milly comes in and restores order to a messy, rambunctious household. My ideal world!

I then checked out about twenty-five more books and headed home.

Back in the olden days when I was a teenager (1981), phones existed, but they were attached to walls by very long cords. The library had such an invention; however, the thought never occurred to me I might want to call and let my dad know I was stopping there and would be late getting home.

I walked into the house to find my dad pacing between the living room and kitchen. His expression was fierce, his eyes wild. He demanded to know where I had been.

I was taken aback by his intensity and mental state; it made me nervous and confused. My complete and utter lack of maturity reared its stupid head, and out of my mouth came a foolish display of bravado. I answered, "What's it to you?"

Yeah.

What transpired after that will not be recounted here. Let's just say it wasn't pretty, and I learned a valuable life lesson that day. I never used that tone or those words with him again, rightfully and respectfully so.

I will tell you now, and have advised my own teenagers to take my example and learn what will *not* gently diffuse the rabid fear parents feel when they are afraid their child might have died or is dying.

My sister had died just months before this interaction with my dad. Because I was not a parent, I didn't have any idea the toll actually having a child die unexpectedly could take, and the possibility something terrible had happened to me wasn't so far-fetched. I didn't put the two together until three months after Emmalynn's funeral.

Emmalynn was conceived and carried and birthed by another woman. I walked into her life knowing her days were limited.

While some of the unknown unsettled us and at times left us a little fearful, we didn't feel terror associated with her dying, because we had already acknowledged that our role was not to save her from death but rather to provide a life.

In December 2012, only a week after our meeting with the foster care social worker, almost everyone in our family had the flu. Mark was pretty much the last man standing. I was down with it; my kids had taken turns puking for days too. The evening of December 20, nineteen-year-old Johanna, ever the responsible one, came into my room and told me I needed to come talk to Emily. She had gotten out of the tub but was not allowing Johanna to help her get dressed.

I fought through the mental fog that the illness had created and thought, *Emily is eleven years old. She does not need you to help her get dressed, seriously.* Irritated, I pulled my aching body up and out of bed and stumbled into Emily's room. She was lying on her bed uncovered, shaking, and most certainly not dressed. What I saw shocked me to complete wakefulness.

Emily appeared to be nearly unconscious; her breathing was loud and deep and labored. Her rib cage was clearly defined. The skin on her collarbones was severely retracted, emphasizing that there was no fat on her chest. Her elbows, knees, and wrists were all sticking out, only skin and bones. Her arms and legs were mottled with lace-like purple discoloration. She was so gaunt that images of concentration camp victims flashed through my head. Fear turned terror gripped my soul. I cried out, gulping with sobs, "Oh my God!"—I was not swearing; I was fervently praying— "Baby girl, what is wrong with you?"

I gathered Emily up in my arms with a blanket wrapped around her and carried her out to the van with the help of Johanna and Charity. I wasn't well myself and obviously not thinking super clearly, since calling 911 would have been the better option. The other kids were sick, so I decided against bringing any of them with me to the hospital. I can't even remember what I told them because my only thought was to get Emily to the hospital as fast as possible. On the way, I got out my flip phone and called Mark, who was at work. In full hysterics I told him to get to the hospital.

Now, when I'm panicked, his first line of defense is to go into super-calm mode (which is super annoying) and land at the opposite end of the emotional spectrum. This kind of response tends to make me feel as though I have to get even more intense to help him understand I'm losing it for a good reason.

He told me in a flat tone, "Calm down. I'm working!"

It was about 9:00 p.m., and he wanted to wait an hour until his shift was over.

Usually I appreciate his work ethic, but in this crisis, it made me so angry my fear was displaced, and I lashed out. "I'm taking Emily to St. Nicholas Hospital!" I took a breath, and before slamming the phone shut, I ended with, *"I. Cannot. Do. This. Alone!"*

I arrived at the hospital and whipped quickly into a parking space. I didn't care if I had parked in between the lines or not. I ran into the building for a wheelchair, zoomed crazily back out again, threw the side door of the van open, and struggled to position Emily in the wheelchair. Then once more I raced like a madwoman into the hospital and pushed Emily straight to the nearby admitting desk, where I am known by sight. (One *benefit* of living in a small town.)

The staff took one look at her, or maybe me, and immediately took us back into the ER, room 4. *Gulp*. Room 4. I knew that room was fully equipped to handle a life-and-death situation. It was the room in which codes were most often called. It was also the room where codes weren't always successful and the patients didn't make it out alive.

Suddenly a flurry of activity broke out, and people rushed past me on all sides. Someone asked me to stand back while the ER team got Emily situated on a gurney. I stood there, trembling almost uncontrollably. I pressed my fist into my mouth to keep from screaming out loud, even though I was certainly doing so in my head.

Emily was very still. Her breathing was ragged, deep, and rasping. Listening to it was agony.

The medical personnel were poking all over her arms trying to get blood for tests. That the poking was unsuccessful was disturbing enough, but even more frightening was Emily's lack of response. She displayed no reaction to the repeated needle sticks, which certainly were causing pain.

The phlebotomist finally got enough blood to send to the lab, and then IV fluids were started. The respiratory therapist applied an oxygen mask to Emily's face, and someone covered her with blankets to warm her mottled, emaciated body.

Throughout those first few minutes, I was hyperventilating and nearly fell down, but somehow I was able to slump into a nearby chair and curl up into the fetal position, dropping my head onto my knees. It was my attempt to slow my breathing and get some blood back to my head.

I heard the nurse tell Emily to slow down her breathing. Sometime later—minutes or hours, I don't know which—the doctor came in and announced, "We've gotten some of her lab results back. Her blood sugars are elevated. She has diabetes."

I choked in disbelief, and my right arm shot up into the air stiff, unyielding. My hand was palm toward him, resisting everything he was saying as if to ward him off and swat him away. I spoke through gritted teeth, my words chopping the air between us in pieces. "No! You do not understand. I don't do diabetes. It's the *flu. SHE HAS THE FLU.* Give her some fluids, and I'm taking her home. She's going to be fine."

After a weighty pause, he quietly said, "She does have the flu. She's also in a ketoacidotic coma. And you do, do diabetes, now." His words were gentle, but they cut me to the core. He was not the enemy, but I felt venomous toward the news he delivered. My fear evaporated, and instead, I felt intensely angry. I was grappling for answers.

I wanted to know why. I wanted to know how. I wanted. . .

My Jesus, I wanted to wake up from this nightmare.

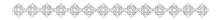

Mark arrived in the room. We were both bewildered, and we paced around in the small space near Emily's bed, hashing through how in the world we had missed the fact that our youngest child had type 1 diabetes. Before Mark had left for work that afternoon, he had told me he had asked Emily to stop hyperventilating. But in my flu-induced stupor, I just thought she was "normal" sick and dismissed it. Shaking our heads in confusion, we were no longer at odds but one in our souls on behalf of our child.

Throughout the winter Emily had worn layers and thick clothing that hid her form. In recent days she had been wearing winter sleepers, which also disguised the dramatic weight loss she had experienced. We knew she was thinner, but it didn't signal an illness because our family's diet had changed due to my celiac disease, and she no longer ate doughnuts, cake, or cookies on a regular basis.

The doctor said the scary hyperventilation she had been doing was actually her body's compensation mechanism, called Kussmaul breathing, which is an effort to preserve life by blowing off CO_2 to offset the metabolic disaster uncontrolled diabetes can cause. This type of breathing signifies the onset of a diabetic coma, and if treatment isn't given, it is the hallmark of imminent death.

We also found out that it's common to discover that a child has diabetes when the flu hits. A diabetic child has a much more debilitating response to illnesses, which often require medical intervention. The mottling on Emily's arms and legs was caused by compromised blood circulation to her limbs—a shutdown—to allow more blood to flow to her organs, keeping her brain and heart, liver, and kidneys functioning. This was another of her body's last-ditch efforts to preserve life. The scariest news, however, was that even with treatment, Emily's brain could swell while she was in the coma, a condition that could be fatal or lead to brain damage.

The ER doctor conferred with the specialist at Children's Hospital in Milwaukee, and they decided that Emily must be moved the sixty miles south to the superior facility. The regular Sheboygan ambulance wasn't sufficiently equipped, and so the move required a pediatric intensive care unit on wheels. The raging blizzard made the road conditions hazardous, but the risk of death from diabetes outweighed the dangers of transporting her to Milwaukee.

Since I was the one who would stay with Emily at Children's Hospital, I needed to go home and get clothing and my purse. Mark stayed with Emily while I went home.

At 2:00 a.m. I began the twenty-seven-block drive while still wearing my pajamas.

I didn't rush. Even if I had wanted to drive recklessly fast, the roads, slick and full of snow, prohibited it and required careful navigation. The streets were empty of traffic. Most people appeared to be at home, snug in their beds, their children sleeping soundly. My thoughts darted to how unfair it was our family had to deal with this, as though somehow we didn't deserve this trouble. As if we had a right to think life is fair.

I felt blindsided by the life-threatening diagnosis of diabetes. My nursing experience had given me compassion toward my patients with the disease but not empathy for the way it turned a world upside down.

I was angry, fuming, yet praying. How crazy is that? I didn't go off on the doctor at the hospital. I did not scream at the nurses about how unfair I felt this was. I went to the One who holds it all.

I found myself screaming and pounding on the steering wheel, crying out in agony, "*You* planned this? Are You kidding me? You planned this? You have messed with me. You have beaten me down. Crushed my heart. Wrecked my physical body so I'll never recover. It is one thing to do it to me, dear God, but how dare You mess with my child! Do you hear me? Not. My. Child!"

My chest heaved out sobs, coughing with the effort, and I felt as if my lungs would explode as I expressed the huge sense of injustice I felt.

The lyrics of "Trust and Obey" flashed through my mind, taking me back to when I sang it with all my might in Sunday school as a child. The pastor's wife pounded away on the old upright piano in the corner of the open basement room. One of the kids held up a large poster with the hymn's words written in huge letters: "Trust and obey, for there's no other way to be happy in Jesus."

Those were sweet words to sing in church on a sunny day in May. On this freezing cold night in December, when the sky was as black as my world, the words mocked me.

Because I was ranting, telling God what I knew to be true from my perspective and not necessarily listening for His take on it, my spirit was not immediately calmed. I didn't have a good explanation for how I could be so adrenalized while at the same time feel beyond exhausted from both the flu and the terror of the past several hours.

Once I arrived at my house, I quickly put on my faded and worn Boy Scout hoodie and jeans, gathered a few other things, and made my way back to the hospital. The trip back had a touch less intensity only because I was completely spent and running on fumes. I reined in my anxious feelings before facing the medical staff in the ER again. When I am afraid, I often feel powerless, and I sometimes flip into angry mode instead, which probably wouldn't accomplish anything worthwhile.

The specialized ambulance and crew arrived from Children's Hospital by 3:00 a.m., and Emily was gently loaded into the back. Two paramedics sat next to her to keep her stable. I was directed up front and climbed wearily into the seat and leaned my head against the icy cold passenger's window, shivering almost uncontrollably.

Mark told me later that he watched as Emily was loaded into the ambulance. His baby was strapped securely on that stretcher, but it may as well have been his own heart. There was nothing he could control or do about it but pray. As the ambulance drove away, he dropped to his knees on the cold driveway, shoulders slumped, and wept.

At Children's Hospital Emily was quickly moved to the ICU, the staff started an insulin drip as well as glucose into Emily's IV lines, and they frequently checked her level of consciousness. "Emily, Emily, do you know where you are?" a doctor or nurse would ask. She gave no response.

Hours later her coma was finally beginning to lift, and one of the doctors came in and did a firm sternal rub, pressing his knuckles hard against her breastbone. This painful stimulus caused her to gasp and tear up.

I gave him an "if looks could kill you'd be ten feet under" scowl; I was not happy at all with his seeming callousness.

Emily stirred slightly, and when he asked again, louder and more insistent this time, "Emily, where are you?" she sighed wearily and said, "I'm. Right. Here."

For the first time in about twenty-four hours, I felt myself smile. She was indeed right here. And if the doctor pressing literally and figuratively didn't know where she was, that was not her problem.

I would like to tell you that God's peace and comfort came in like a flood and carried me away on a life raft of love. It didn't happen like that. No audible voice or quiet inner voice assured me all was going to be well. I simply placed one foot in front of the other, having no ability to see down the road and not knowing for sure that anything would ever be all right again.

Ironically, I had faith that God was listening to my prayers even though I hissed some of them. I knew God was real even if it seemed as though He wasn't helping me. I couldn't be angry with Someone who didn't exist, could I? I would have drowned in hopelessness and been completely lost if I couldn't pray through my anger. Warm and fuzzy would not describe our relationship in that moment. Deep down I felt steady and secure, knowing He was hearing me, whether or not He was answering in a way I liked. Praying helped me to avoid panicking and kept me at the level of just plain ol' mad.

Preachers had warned me that being angry with or disappointed in God was wrong because He always did everything right and good.

And so He does.

But I had also read about a hundred different psalms where the writer cried out in anger, despair, sadness, or bewilderment. "Where are You, God?" the psalmists lamented. "And why are You so far from helping me?" At that time, those were the types of questions I was praying.

I realized there had to be a difference between blaspheming God (taunting His justice and questioning His character) and crying out in despair. I felt that my brutal honesty was a sincere offering. He knew my thoughts already, so how in the world could I fake a happy face and good attitude?

I felt as if it had to be okay not to be okay.

Emily eventually came out of the coma. I should have been ecstatic, but I was still numb. She was then moved to the eleventh floor, which is for stabler patients. The doctors and nurses hit us with an onslaught of information about insulin dosages and glucose parameters and how to operate a meter and how to detect dangerous blood sugar levels, and on and on. It was too much to take in. I was walking around dazed and numb. There didn't seem to be any time to process our grief over the loss of health and what we considered a normal life. Instead, we had to get with the program and learn how to treat her diabetes.

"Mama," she said, "I can't wait to get out of here. I don't want any more shots." This broke my heart because to live she had to have several daily insulin injections. I gently gave the news to her that the shots were the new normal.

"I'm not going to eat; then I won't have to have insulin." She was grasping at possibilities other than the ones presented by the medical staff. It was a nice thought but not realistic.

When I had taken our first child home from the hospital and realized she didn't come with a manual, I had felt inadequate and uncertain. But that was nothing compared to the feelings of trepidation when we drove Emily home from the hospital. I knew her meds or her food could get messed up in any number of ways and she might die as a result. But I could not lie down on the floor and give in to the fear. For her sake I had to be braver than I was, and had to choose to act how I wished I felt.

Those first days back at home were dark. We had more questions than answers. To help us understand the diabetes lifestyle, six of us took classes at the Children's Hospital clinic building. Emily and I took a second course to make sure we comprehended the disease and its nuances. Isn't the first rule of battle to know your enemy? Well, this enemy was crafty.

I really, really like walking into chaos and having the ability to restore order. Diabetes, however, can only be relatively controlled. For example, let's say Emily did x, y, and z in one twenty-four hour period, and she subsequently had great blood sugar readings. The next day she could do x, y, and z in exactly the same way and her sugars could be out of range. The unpredictability of hormones, food, lack of sleep, excess sleep, exercise, cold temperatures, and stress could affect her body's ability to utilize the insulin injected into her arms, legs, or belly. And if she got ill, oh boy, that could be a wild ride. This blood-sugar roller coaster would result in many tearful moments.

"I don't want to live with this disease, Mom," she told me one day. "I just can't. It's too much. It's never going away. I'm never going to get better. How am I supposed to do this for the *rest of my life*?"

Emily's question and others like it have driven me to pray like I have not done on my own behalf. I don't have trite answers; if I did go down that path, she would blow those off quicker than I could say them. The response I usually give is "You don't have to do this for the rest of your life today. You don't even have to do tomorrow today. Just get through this next minute or two."

I dreaded and feared the day she would get ill and the "Sick Day" protocol would kick in. And because God is good, that fear was faced head-on. The day came when it had to be instituted. Emily had the stomach flu again, not terrible, but enough that she couldn't keep any food down. A normal child can go twenty-four hours without eating or drinking. They'll be shaky but okay. For a diabetic there is no such luxury as waiting it out. You don't say, "Toughen up and you'll be fine." At the very least she had to be able to keep down sugary liquids so she could receive insulin. She tossed everything back up again in spite of having antinausea medicine. Finally, after a day of checking Emily's glucose levels every hour, the heavy uncertainty of whether I was doing the best thing or not, and making multiple phone calls to update the diabetes nurse, we cried uncle. We couldn't manage the vomiting at home and had to go to the hospital. She was given IV fluids and glucose, and then was able to be given insulin injections.

What I had feared and dreaded and made me pray, "Oh God, please not that," had happened. And crazy enough, the days moving forward became more doable because the scariness of the unknown was relieved. We then knew what we could manage at home and what would require a trip to the hospital. Once we had faced and conquered another worst-case scenario, the fear of the unknown had another bite taken out of it.

But my responses to Emily's sugars being too low or too high unsettled my daughter. My heart being clenched in a tight fist of fear over the possibility she could die tainted almost all of our interactions. This inability on my part to let go of my need to control her disease nearly killed her because of her intense desire not to worry me.

I was suddenly up close and personal to the very real potential of having one of my own biological children die, and my fears about it had to be shaken and overcome. I found comfort in these verses from Hebrews 2:14–15: "By embracing death, taking it into himself, he destroyed the Devil's hold on death and freed all who cower through life, *scared to death of death*" (MSG, emphasis added).

On December 28, 2013, our family celebrated Mary Elisabeth's sixteenth birthday. Dozens of friends packed inside the house. It was part of the kids' normal chaotic after-Christmas sledding party. Boots, hats, gloves, wet coats, and snowy mud tracks littered the first floor of our home. The hungry sledders chowed down pancakes and sipped hot chocolate. A fire blazed in the fireplace. The music was cranked up. The kids played games, talked, and lounged all over the family room, kitchen, dining and living rooms. There were bodies, bodies everywhere.

I was busy staying on top of the food supply and washing the dishes piling up all over the house. I don't know whether I asked Emily what her sugars were that day, but I assumed since we had a year in of blood-sugar management, she was probably fine. This was an assumption I should not have made.

At 3:00 a.m. Mark and I awoke to a loud banging on the wall between our bedroom and Emily's. We'd had no experience with this kind of noise before; it was rhythmic and repetitive. Mark called out her name, but she didn't answer. I threw off the blankets and dashed across the room saying, "Dear God! I think she's seizing!"

Mark stopped briefly to throw on a pair of pants before running to get to Emily. In the five seconds it took to get out of our door and into her room and flip on the light, the noise hadn't abated. We found her writhing in bed, limbs flailing everywhere. Her head was repeatedly hitting the wall and the desk.

Mark instantly dropped to his knees by her low platform bed. I shouted as I headed down the hall, "Turn her on her left side so she doesn't choke on her vomit! I'll call 911!"

I ran down the stairs—half tripping in my haste—and flipped on the light in the dining room. I grabbed the phone with hands shaking so badly I could hardly dial the number. "C'mon! C'mon! C'mon!" I said over and over to myself. "Dang it all; get your fingers to work!"

The 911 operator answered quickly, and I explained our emergency. She said she would send the EMTs to our home.

I then glanced to my right and saw several pairs of eyes staring at me! I realized I was standing there in my underwear and a T-shirt. The youths observing my harried actions and hearing my frantic words were Joshua's friends from New Tribes Bible Institute who had come up to go sledding the day before.

Hello!

I put up my right hand toward them, shaking my head no, as if to say, "I cannot deal with you right now. I am so sorry you're seeing me like this, but in the whole scheme of things, I don't care!"

I ran around in the dining room to flip on the Christmas lights to illuminate our porch and front door, which I unlocked, and I ran back upstairs to Mark, who had been frantically calling me to come help him. As frightening as it was, there wasn't much to do for Emily but try to keep her from hurting herself. Mark was sitting behind her back, propping her on her left side, both to keep her from aspirating any vomit but also to aid in some small way any breathing efforts she might be trying to make. Keeping her arms and legs and head from banging into the wall or the desk was the best we could do in the moment. I had glucagon but was too freaked out even to put two thoughts together to get it mixed up and injected. I felt like the worst mom ever. The grand mal seizures were contorting her features. Her hair was long, but stringy and coated in vomit, plastered in places to her forehead and neck. It was distressing to watch. I stepped quickly into my bedroom to throw on a pair of sweats so the paramedics didn't have to deal with my state of undress. (No use in scaring or scarring them, too.)

The rest of the household was awake and congregated downstairs wondering what in the world was happening. Andrew, at thirteen years old, always the gentleman and naturally stepping into the role of directing traffic, met the Sheboygan Fire Department truck and ambulance with their EMTs and sent them upstairs to Emily's room. She ended up being transported to St. Nicholas Hospital again.

We later learned her blood sugars had dropped to un-detectable levels and then too low to manage anywhere except at a hospital. The grand mal seizures had developed because her brain needed glucose. All the shaking of her muscles was to release any sugar in them, get it into her bloodstream and then to her brain and vital organs. God has made our bodies fearfully and wonderfully and built in ways for life to be preserved in spite of seriously adverse circumstances.

Emily was in the emergency room for a couple of hours while we waited to be admitted.

I would need to be at her side to help maintain her health and safety, in spite of my feelings of complete in-adequacy to manage her diabetes. Once again I ran home to get some clothing for myself while Mark remained with Emily in the ER.

I got home and lay down for a minute on my bed. I wasn't ranting and raving; instead, the tears dripped silently out of the outside corners of my eyes and into my hair and ears. I just wanted to catch my breath and decompress for a second before heading back to the hospital where I had to be strong. I could not fall apart emotionally. My reprieve was short-lived, cut off by my ringing phone. I answered to find our personal pediatrician, and friend, was on the line. "Hey! Dr. T here!" he said. "When are you coming back? Your husband is not being very helpful." He clipped his sentences out in his signature short-and-direct fashion, not necessarily waiting for a response to the first question before asking another.

I laughed so hard the tears started again. I could imagine the two of them attempting to communicate about medical things. I assured him I would be back very shortly.

I arrived at the ER, didn't see Dr. T, and asked Mark what was up.

He told me, "Dr. T came in and said, 'I need to know your kids' names, their birthdates, and their health history.' I told him, 'I know my kids' names—all eight of them—not necessarily in order. I do not know their birthdates, and I definitely don't know their health history. That's my wife's job!' and then he walked out."

After the night's emotional roller coaster, this no-nonsense, prefers-to-remain-ignorant approach my husband takes (and makes no apology for) provided me with some much-needed, though brief, comic relief.

My fear over feeling responsible to keep my child alive threatened to consume me. What I hadn't known was that Emily had a dilemma about dosing with insulin. She had met many a type 2 diabetic in our social circles who told her they didn't have to check their sugars with a painful finger poke. They just knew by the way they felt that their sugar was high. They also didn't need insulin injections. They took a pill. They misunderstood the vast difference between the type 2 diabetes they had and Emily's type 1, which affects only 5 to 10 percent of the diabetes population. This misinformation left Emily believing the doctors and I had lied to her about how to manage her disease. Why was she the only one who had to get stuck with needles all the time? Why couldn't she just swallow a pill when she felt a little off?

At bedtime the night before, she assumed her sugars were probably very high because of all the syrup and cocoa she had consumed at the party. She misread the dial on her insulin pen and accidentally took thirty units of insulin, which is about six times what she normally takes. She then realized her mistake, checked her blood sugar—which was normal—and decided to go eat a bunch more junk food to help elevate her blood glucose. She told me later, "No way, no how did I want to come tell you at 10:00 p.m. what I'd done and have you freak out about it." This wasn't a sound decision on her part, but her fear of my reaction was greater than her fear of her actions. I have already described the fallout of this decision. She learned a sober lesson about the difference between type 1 and type 2 diabetes, and it was a valuable one. She's a walking miracle. God definitely has a plan for her life because, humanly speaking, *she should not still be here.*

Emily is a treasure and similar to me in personality. We're both "pistols," passionate and enthusiastic. This makes for some heated exchanges. Remember the sassy attitude I had toward my dad when I got home late after staying at the library? Emily has come home late a few times from the library, too, a perfectly acceptable place to go, but not when no one has any idea she's going there instead of coming straight home from school. I have not exercised the self-control I should have when she seems unwilling to manage her diabetes carefully or to let me know where she is at all times. This can create anxiety in my mother-heart. I have allowed her unexplained absences and then her snarky responses to my inquiries to take my wild fear for her well-being and turn it into anger.

I have sat on Emily's bed and asked for forgiveness because my angry response to her was not justified, even though her behavior needed correction. My fear has been a lack of faith that God has her in hand and cares much more for her well-being here on earth and eternally than I ever could, and while that is hard to imagine, it is nevertheless true.

Emily's days are numbered, and they were before there was even one of them. God knew her in my womb and knitted her body together exactly as He wanted it to be. Nothing that has happened in her life has taken Him by surprise. He is in control, and He is accomplishing His will. God has graciously preserved my life. He has preserved my daughter's life on more than one occasion. For example, the night Emily was diagnosed with diabetes, Johanna had been prompted in her heart several times to go upstairs and put some lotion on Emily's legs. This isn't strange, as Emily has always had very dry skin, but Johanna didn't want to go. She wasn't feeling well, and Emily's legs could wait for another day, but the thought that she should get up and go to Emily persisted. After going to Emily's room, when she started to apply the lotion, she was confused and frightened to find that her sister's legs were like sticks they were so thin. The skin was waxy white and looked like she was wearing purple lace nylon stockings because of the circulation being compromised to both her arms and legs. Johanna had no idea how sick Emily was, but the appearance of her lower limbs and her unwillingness to allow Johanna to get her dressed and warm caused her to come find me. Emily would have died very soon afterward in her bed alone if Johanna had not followed the promptings to check on her. On the day she had the grand mal seizures, if she had been farther down in her bed, her head would not have hit the wall between our bedrooms. Mark and I were deep in sleep and might not have heard any noise. So she once again could have easily died, and we would not have known until morning.

"Death in bed" syndrome is a real thing for diabetics. One way that we handle it is to ask in the morning, "Has anybody talked to Emily today? Is she still breathing?" We're not kidding. The words are said calmly as though we have asked whether someone wants eggs or oatmeal for breakfast, but we don't let the light tone in which they are said take away from the seriousness of the inquiry.

I have had to learn to trust that God intensely loves and is carrying Emily, and is carrying us, no matter what happens. At times I have chosen to believe otherwise, and I have been heck to live with and made everybody miserable, dying "a thousand deaths dreading one."[1]

She told me the other day, "You know, Mom, it's kind of crazy what used to freak us out, and now you're like '*Pfft*, your sugar's 450, what are you doing about it?' and you're not panicked anymore. All the stuff that was so scary just isn't that big of a deal." We're not lighthearted with a careless attitude toward the danger Emily could be in, but the stranglehold that fear has had on my heart has lessened and in turn helped my daughter, who can be more scared by my response to her diabetes than by the disease itself.

I have gone through the Esther study by Beth Moore[2] a number of times, and the material helped me put things into perspective. Satan has threatened me time and again over the years, causing fear to well up and seize my heart and mind over the possibility that one of my children could die unexpectedly. "Is God good," he taunts, "if He lets that happen?" I consciously choose over and over again (not just once and done), not to live there, being threatened and thinking to myself that I could declare God unjust and unfair because He didn't answer my prayers the way I wanted, that I could rail against heaven, declaring God unloving should one of my kids die.

Honestly, I have to go there. Bottom line, the worst fears in my life have to do with being disabled and death, so I process each fear as it rises. If this ___ (fill in the worst-case scenario), then God. Then God. Then God. I'm not able to flutter about, thinking, *Oh, that could never happen, so don't even worry about it.*

For me it's not enough to trust God that it won't happen; I have to trust Him *even if it does.* God is good, and He loves me despite the circumstances. Knowing this carries me through the valley of the shadow of death and helps me not to be overcome with fear of evil. To me, faith means I might not understand how God is working all things together for good and for His glory when they appear so terrible, but He is. This knowledge steadies me when my world seems to be falling apart.

I don't know what the future holds. What I know to be true is this: My God brings beauty from ashes. My God is faithful. He does what He pleases, and it will all be worked together for the ultimate good, whether it is in the moment or not. I can trust Him with my own life and with my children's lives.

I firmly believe one of the ways God redeemed my thinking and actions through Emily's diabetes was to give me an understanding of parents who find themselves unable to continue to care for their children. It helps me put aside any pride and offer compassion to those who have made the choice to put their children in foster care or had the choice made for them.

When I first began to deal with Emily's diagnosis and grappled with my responsibilities, I found myself wishing I could drop her off at Children's Hospital and let her stay there as if it were some kind of boarding school. She would be kept safe and medically cared for. I would promise to visit her, of course! Then we would marry her off to Superman when she was twenty-three years old, and he would make sure from then on that she was okay. Let someone else much better equipped handle it, because I felt totally inept and afraid.

This fear made my child a little crazy. If I was as old as I was and so afraid of diabetes, how could she, at eleven years old, live with it without dreading each day? God, because He is faithful, has carried and kept both Emily and me through this storm, and we are not the same people today as we were back in 2012. We are more aware of and empathetic toward the suffering around us. God has continued to educate and equip us to handle the trial He has asked us to bear.

9

BREATH OF LIFE

I surrender all,
I surrender all.
All to Thee, my blessed Savior,
I surrender all.

—JUDSON W. VAN DEVENTER, "I SURRENDER ALL"

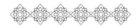

Life is not a paved, smooth road with a straight trajectory. The same is true of foster care.

During the vetting of potential foster parents, a candidate can easily miss the mark. Here are the portions Mark and I had finished.

> Psych evaluation passed ☑
> Education requirements completed ☑
> Personal interviews approved ☑
> References verified ☑

We found this process to be deterring at times yet also reassuring. A kiddo's well-being and safety shouldn't be compromised while in foster care. The agency Mark and I work with goes above and beyond to ensure success on the part of all involved. We are honored to be part of the system.

In early 2013 we were given the final approval to become licensed medical treatment foster parents. The soul struggle over having others scrutinize my life—all our lives—was real. God had begun a good work of establishing my worth apart from my abilities, and He continued it during the season of waiting for word that the Salchert family was indeed competent to care for children.

And then the wait began in earnest.

One year after our licensing was completed, we finally received a call about a child who was actually going to be placed with our family. A real live baby was placed in our arms and our home.

When he first came to us, his brows had a permanent crease. He looked like an old man with too many worries. He had been pretty miserable his first few weeks. He wasn't terminally ill, but rather his medical challenges required our nurturing. With seven sets of open arms at our house, Baby B was held most of the time, which was helpful in soothing his anxieties. He grew into a beautiful, happy, smiling, giggling baby. He was going to be adopted by biological relatives, and we were gifted with the ability to get to know his family before he transitioned to live with them.

We poured out our hearts, giving that baby boy tons of love and cuddling in the eight months he was with us. We treated him as though he were going to live with us forever, no matter how long his stay. No regrets.

My fervent prayer was that I would be able to give Baby B over to his adoptive mother's arms and do so with a smile so that the last time he saw me, my face wouldn't be a mess because I was crying. God answered abundantly above what I requested, and Baby B grinned at me in a way that assured me he was going to be better than okay, and eventually so was I.

I came home from the journey to give Baby B up on

my birthday, September 28, 2014, resolved that I was done fostering—at least for a while. I felt as if my heart was broken even though it was a *good* thing that had transpired. We had done a wonderful job where our foster baby was concerned. Also, Johanna, our oldest daughter still at home, was in the process of gathering support to go live and work at an orphanage in Thailand. I wanted to make sure she had the time and energy to dedicate to that effort.

Mark, on the other hand, had a different perspective. He told me about a week later, "You need to call the social worker. Get back in the saddle."

"No, I want time to heal," I explained. "I miss the baby so badly. I wake up in the morning imagining I hear him playing in his crib and giggling, but then I realize he's not really there." I shook my head, not wanting to open myself up to having my heart broken—again and on purpose.

"Nope. This is what you do. Give her a call," was Mark's summation of the situation.

The following weekend Mark was driving the van, which was packed with all our kids currently living with us. I turned around in my seat so I could see all of them and asked, "What do you think about getting another baby? Dad says I should call our social worker and let her know. I have no idea how soon we would get a child. But I do know we all miss Baby B and are hurting, so if you're not up for it yet, that's perfectly okay."

I wanted to accurately evaluate their responses. Everyone in the van nodded yes, from Charity, Johanna, Emily, and Andrew. Mary Elisabeth, who was seventeen at the time, told me flat out, "Uh, Mom, what if some kid needs us and you're just sitting over here with a broken heart?"

I turned back around, facing the front window. I smiled

and thought, *Okay, fine. I'll call Faith.*

I called the next morning. And not too many days after that we were asked if we would take a four-month-old boy named Charlie who was in the ICU at Children's Hospital. Faith told us he had a tracheostomy (breathing tube), and we didn't know much more than that.

Johanna, Charity, and I drove to the hospital to meet the little one.

People with dreamy smiles have asked me this question, "Oh, did you just fall in love with him right away?"

Nope, I didn't.

He was a sorry sight when we arrived in the room. He was upset and posturing, which means his head was arched backward, his body stiff. With his blotchy, red skin, honestly, he was one of the most unattractive babies I had ever seen.

I washed my hands and asked if I could hold him in my arms and close to me so it would be easier to look him over. My desire to look him over closely was in no way to evaluate his cuteness factor and decide if we wanted him or not. The decision had already been made sight unseen. I was fact finding, not fault finding.

I pulled up one of the hospital recliners next to his bed, and the nurse detangled the tubes and wires that monitored his heart rate and his oxygen saturations. The long blue tubing delivering humidified air to his tracheostomy had to be juggled to get him into my lap.

My heart quailed inside me at the sight of all this equipment attached to him. He needed all that just to keeping him going! *Wow.*

When he was settled in my lap, as much as a stiff, unhappy child could be, I realized his eyes were rolled back in his head. The heaviness of that moment bowled over me like a semitruck. I thought, *There is a baby underneath all this equipment. Don't forget that, Salchert.*

"He is profoundly brain-damaged," I said flatly to the nurse. It wasn't a question.

"Yes, he is."

My breath caught in my chest, and I consciously exhaled, absorbing the shock.

In seconds I processed the great responsibility we were taking on. The decision to care for this child had not been made lightly, and that resolve stabilized me. Charlie reminded me so much of my little sister, Amie. While Amie hadn't had an artificial airway, the way they both had seizures and spasticity—eyes rolled back in their heads, unseeing—brought my childhood memories to the forefront.

I gave myself an internal pep talk: *You always wanted to be able to do more for Amie. You're an adult now. You have nursing skills. You couldn't do very much for your sister, but you could make a difference for this baby.*

I made a decision to act based on how I wanted to feel. I didn't have a rush of adoring love for him initially, but compassion? Oh, you betcha.

It was also Johanna's twenty-first birthday, so we regrouped at The Cheesecake Factory a couple of miles from the hospital. I was quiet during lunch, reflecting on all we had seen in Charlie's hospital room and how much we were expected to learn in a short time frame.

The rule was that two people over the age of eighteen years old had to be able to completely take care of all of his needs. Charity was in nursing school and the natural choice for the position, but she had schedule restraints, as did Mark, who was still working full-time.

Johanna became my go-to, the second caregiver required to bring Charlie home. She was planning to go back to Thailand permanently as a missionary but had to raise support in the States to pay for her room and board. Those funds hadn't come in yet, so she was at home and willing to step up and help for the short term.

Johanna and I stayed the night close to the hospital—one lousy, awful, noisy night in an inexpensive hotel. The room was dirty even though, for some odd reason, the staff ran the vacuum cleaner up and down the halls at 3:00 a.m.!

The next day as we sat in Charlie's room in the ICU, I shook my head in some confusion and said, "I don't know how we're going to spend six weeks down here to learn how to competently care for this baby."

Could we travel back and forth a couple of hours every day? We couldn't afford to stay in a hotel night after night, and with my dietary restrictions, food was another crazy hurdle. As the impossibilities loomed large, I asked myself, *Did we miss it? This is not doable. Physically, I can't fall apart in the process of trying to take care of this baby.* I was a little confused at how hard the process was turning out to be.

My phone rang. A staff member of the Ronald McDonald House was on the line. The house was across the street from the hospital and provided lodging for families whose children were in the hospital or receiving long-term outpatient treatment. She said they had a room for us that night if we wanted it and for as long as we might need it. Johanna urged me to go ahead and take it. We got settled in and found the impossibilities that faced us were lifted in one fell swoop.

We would come back in the evenings after spending

hours with Charlie, famished and tired, not just physically but on every front. Most of the time a meal had been lovingly prepared for us. The food was nourishing, not just for our bodies but also for our souls, making us feel cherished.

Our home-away-from-home at the Ronald McDonald House was a safe haven in the midst of the storm. I felt nurtured and cared for by the kindhearted, benevolent efforts of others who had no idea who we were but gave generously anyway. That kindness had a way of getting paid forward to the people who came across my path, especially our foster son.

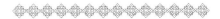

Charlie required surgery not too long after we became his foster family. A feeding tube, called a G-J, was placed in his abdomen and routed nourishment through his stomach into his small intestine. Before this, like Emmalynn, he had been fed through a small tube that entered his nose.

His recovery period after the surgery was rough. He wasn't bothering to breathe on his own, and a ventilator was brought to his aid.

This change in Charlie's health status, combined with the pressure of learning how to use a new piece of vital and complicated equipment, knocked me for a loop. Charlie wasn't initially considered terminal, though his prognosis was poor. He occasionally didn't have respiratory drive when he fell asleep, and so his oxygen saturations would drop. He couldn't stay awake all the time, and expecting someone to watch him like a hawk should he stop breathing was just as unrealistic—and yet we tried it. At first we thought if we were holding him, we would certainly notice if his breathing stopped. But he didn't wave his hands in the air and announce, "I will now stop breathing." No, the little dude would be lying in our arms, his skin color sweet and pink one minute, and the next we would look down and he would be gray. This would happen without any fanfare or warning. There was no discernible cause for this other than the oxygen shortages he had experienced in the womb and at birth (called hypoxic-ischemic encephalopathy).

This was my first rodeo with a child this medically fragile. Charlie was what is called a "full code." (Resuscitation measures are a gift for most people, and for some, in my opinion, they are not.) Everything must be done to save his life, including introducing air into his lungs via a respiratory bag or ventilator and applying compressions of his sternum and ribcage to pump blood through his heart. These compressions could certainly result in his sternum cracking or his ribs being broken, which would cause him great pain. "Full code" also includes using a defibrillator and injecting cardiac meds in his veins or via the space inside his bones should IV access not be available. All this was hanging over him—and us. He was oblivious to the potential outcomes, but we were not. It was a heavy, almost suffocating, burden to bear on his behalf.

One evening I went back to the Ronald McDonald House and went to the dining room on the third floor. I sat on a chair in the corner of the room. I was trying to get some supper because it had been hours since my last meal, and I couldn't seem to pull myself together. I called my husband and wept over the phone.

The room was empty except for Elsie, one of the cleaning ladies. I was focused on the phone call and not paying attention to her as she worked. I questioned Mark. "I don't know if we're supposed to do this. It's so hard. Did we miss it? Do I want the redemption of the loss I felt over Amie so badly that I have taken on something I should not be doing?"

Mark wasn't experiencing any doubts in that moment and said, "I don't think God changed His mind about all of this just because it's tougher than we realized it was going to be. We believed it was what we should do a few weeks ago. He hasn't decided we shouldn't do it now and forgot to send the memo."

Elsie came over to my table. She placed a tissue box, a couple of granola bars, and a bottle of water in front of me. Without a word, she gently reached out, placed her hand on my shoulder, and gave it a little squeeze. I looked up, and she nodded her head in my direction with a wink, as if to say, "You've got this." Then she moved away without saying anything and went back to her work.

At one of the care conferences, which is a meeting to evaluate our readiness for taking Charlie home, one of the nurse practitioners said, "Oh, you're so cute. Look at how scared you are." I didn't necessarily feel cute at all. It was one thing to care for Charlie in the hospital where there was a call light. If it went off, at a moment's notice, nurses, doctors, respiratory therapists, care partners, and/or equipment maintenance people would come running. At home *we were it*. All those jobs wrapped up in two shaky humans who cared a lot but could make a mistake and kill this child as a result.

I had never liked working with NICU babies. The hospice ones, yes—my ability to make a difference (and not cause harm) was pretty much guaranteed. I felt confident in that arena. Charlie, however, was not supposed to come home and die. We had to do our best to prevent mistakes.

I tried my best to be educated and competent to care for any baby in the nursery while I worked on the labor and delivery floor, but situations with babies in critical need where I was the one primarily in charge were not ones I relished or enjoyed. Now I had a choice to master the skills to care well for Charlie and not let fear have its way, or I could leave him at the hospital and say, "Nope, I'm not going there."

We had been told our "deer in the headlights" look would vanish after a while and we would pack up his Go-bag, a term used for the bag that kids with a tracheostomy who are on ventilators have with them 24/7 with all the tracheostomy supplies and the resuscitation bag. I also had to manage his diaper bag, the wheelchair, ventilator, and pulse oximeter, not to mention the boy himself. They said it would become so routine that we would wonder what we were ever so fearful about. The transition from acute fear to "*pfft*, whatever" took a long time with many, many bumps in the road.

Caitlin, one of the nurses in the ICU, took on the bulk of the responsibility to teach Johanna and me how to do what was called "Charlie's cares."

One of my first bumps was on the morning I needed to do his first trach tube change. All the supplies were carefully laid out on the bedside table. I had read the procedure steps a number of times. I had watched it being done. I had practiced on a little red *Sesame Street* Elmo doll.

As I stood at Charlie's bedside, his tiny new trach in my shaking gloved hand, I felt my knees go weak. Caitlin was on the other side of the bed and said, "Are you okay? I'm right here. I know what to do if he gets into trouble. You're not alone. I'll walk you through step by step."

This was good to hear, but for heaven's sake, I wasn't able to convince my heart to believe it.

She observed my continued hesitation—and perhaps the paralyzed look on my face—and motioned to put the trach back in the container. I did so, stepping back from the bed. I found the chair with the back of my knees and dropped into it with a choking sob.

Caitlin was fabulous. In no way did she downplay my fear; she didn't make fun of it or tell me it was irrational. She just asked what I was thinking.

I told her with my voice quavering, "*I don't want to hurt him*. If I don't get this trach in correctly, he cannot breathe. I'm not sure I can be what he needs."

The nurse didn't immediately tell me, "You loser." And she didn't flippantly answer with "You can't hurt him." Because neither was true.

She did tell me I didn't have to do any of it right then, but she didn't leave in a huff as though I couldn't do it. She simply let me catch my breath and waited with anticipation and confidence, which assured me that I could handle it.

I contemplated within the space of a minute or two what was at stake if I chose to let fear intimidate me. It was not a little red doll lying in the bed in front of me, but a live child, making removing and replacing an artificial but oh-so-necessary airway more difficult, but the baby under all those wires and tubes would be left simply to exist in the hospital if I focused solely on his equipment.

I stood up, and with my jaw firmly set, told Caitlin, "Let's try this again."

And we did it.

And I did not hurt him.

Getting the first trach change out of the way was the hardest. The mental and emotional hurdle I had to jump was done, and Charlie was okay. Fear took a huge hit that day, and I do believe the heavens cheered.

Fear had to continue taking a backseat as time progressed. The training Johanna and I received was completed by December, and we brought Charlie home in time for Christmas.

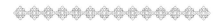

What Charlie most needed from us was to be treated affectionately and to have his medical cares competently addressed. In chatting with my kids, none of us remembers initially having overwhelming feelings of love for him. Instead, we were mostly terrified because of his breathing issues. It was a decision of our wills to treat him as if we loved him until the emotion joined our actions.

Charlie needs someone with him 24/7 because of his potential airway obstruction issues. This means we have a couple of nurses who help so we can get other things done to maintain our household and care for the rest of the family members. One thing one of our day nurses did was to pull Charlie into her lap and turn on her iPod. She placed one ear bud in her ear and the other in Charlie's. He appeared to relax and enjoy being snuggled like this, and I encouraged her to spend as much time as possible holding him, not simply doing his meds or suctioning. She was more than willing to comply. Another of our day nurses likes to watch *Andy Griffith* reruns with Charlie lying against her chest so he can see the screen, and she reads in an animated way to him all the time. Charlie wiggles his way into his favorite comfortable position on her lap and enjoys the stroking she does along his neck and behind his ear as they watch the Kindle. He doesn't register any response to medical tests for vision or hearing, but he most definitely sees his toys above his bed, because he hits them with his fist with amazing accuracy.

I requested a regular-sized hospital bed for quality-of-life reasons. I realized my husband and Andrew were not holding Charlie. They were too afraid of disrupting his equipment to pick him up out of the crib by themselves, and they didn't want to hassle with taking the time to get him all detangled and settled in the chair and then have to put him back to bed fairly quickly because the guys have "no sit in them."

The hospital bed allows anyone to climb in and lay next to Charlie and be as close as they would like without having to move any of his wires or tubing. The little man is hilarious to lie next to. You'll think he's sleeping or oblivious, but as soon as you lie down next to him, his left hand comes up and he will repeatedly stroke your face or smack you until you hold his hand and talk to him. He is not content to lie quietly; he wants your full attention and will badger you until he gets it!

One of Charlie's favorite things is being taken outside in his wheelchair or stroller. When he first started riding around in his stroller, there was an umbrella over the top of it. He swung both of his arms back to knock the canopy out of the way so he could see. I put the canopy back again, thinking it was a fluke, but he did it again. Once more I put the canopy back, and the little booger knocked it out of his way every single time until I finally took it off completely. Because of Charlie's vision issues, he stares at the sun and doesn't blink, squint, or otherwise protect his eyes, so we have to put sunglasses on him. He wouldn't put up with the stroller canopy, but he tolerates the glasses with a better attitude.

I live by faith somewhat in interpreting Charlie's needs because he is unable to communicate verbally. He typically doesn't make eye contact, and his eyes don't light up with recognition or joy even when they are focused. Our knowledge of him and he of us is much more intangible.

Taking a baby to a well-child checkup at Dr. T's office was a familiar adventure for him and me. Dr. T remembered when I had brought Emmalynn to see him in the office. The nurse that August day asked me to get her undressed, weighed her, and told me Dr. T was supposed to be right in to examine Emmalynn. He got delayed and took longer than expected. I let Emmalynn lie there on the examining table only a minute or two, and then, because I didn't want to redress her, I pulled up my T-shirt and tucked her in against my tummy, leaving only her little head exposed in the crook of my arm. I was swaying back and forth humming when Dr. T came in and saw us. He shook his head and said, "You've gotten attached haven't you?" All I could say very quietly was, "That ship sailed for sure," meaning I had indeed fallen in love with that sweet baby. My instinct to keep her warm and protected was in full mama-bear mode. I hadn't given birth to Emmalynn, but I loved her as if I had.

When I held Charlie so Dr. T could examine him, he saw I had once again fallen head over heels in love with a baby destined to eventually break my heart.

"You're nuts! You know that?" he said.

"Yep, probably, but I can't stand the thought of this kiddo dying in the hospital alone without a family. I'm not expecting you to cure him or fix him. I just need a right-hand man up here in Sheboygan, and you're it!"

Dr. T has taken care of my kids for years, and in spite of his misgivings, he has trusted my judgment and heart enough to continue making house calls when needed, and he puts up with my craziness.

Other health care workers have also supported us in caring for Charlie. One of the most encouraging things a hospital nurse said to me was this: "You know, we can tell when kiddos are cared for and when they are neglected. The parents say they are doing things for their baby, and because the kids can't tell us any differently, the parents think we don't know what's really going on. Charlie is obviously loved, and you're doing a great job of meeting his physical needs." Those words affirmed our actions of holding him, bathing him, applying lotion, and massaging his little body. His skin was in excellent shape as a result. His ability to relax was testimony to the fact he trusted us and was pain-free. In the day-to-day business of caring for his needs, those small, loving actions can look inconsequential. What a sweet thing to find out all that mundane stuff added up and made his existence not only bearable but also enjoyable.

In June 2015 the foster care social workers asked Mark and me about our thoughts on adopting Charlie. Life had certainly been chaotic in the six months we'd had him home. He had been hospitalized on several occasions, and he had come close to death too many times to count. My prayers that God would give me a deep love for this sweet baby had been answered, and I had no desire for him to live somewhere else or with anyone else.

The ramifications of making Charlie a permanent part of our family were heavy, and we considered our options carefully. If we adopted him, Mark and I were not sure we would be able to financially provide for him. Some of those concerns were allayed when we found out that his health insurance would continue and that we would be given some assistance to offset the extra expenses even after we legally made him our child. As he grew older, however, we would incur expenses that would not be covered.

As a result of my disabling surgeries, I was not working and bringing in a paycheck. I do not get paid to be a mom.

One of my fears in life—a dragon I have had to slay repeatedly—is the fear of looking stupid. I do my best to be informed so events don't sneak up on me and leave me in a bind. So before we agreed to adopt Charlie, I thought through everything as best as I could. Adopting Charlie meant we might have to have a wheelchair accessible van, a ramp into the house, and a hydraulic lift to pick him up because he would get heavier as he grew. His spasticity can be difficult to manage and difficult to contain. If he's lying in my lap but doesn't like that position anymore, he stiffens. He's also dead weight when being held because he has low muscle tone (called hypotonia), so he isn't able to make any effort to bear his own weight by wrapping his arms or legs around my neck or waist. Moreover, I hadn't made time to work out in years, so the muscles in my arms, back, and legs were weaker than I liked.

We could not afford a van or renovations in the house to accommodate Charlie's growing needs, and we did not want to put our family in a place where we would accrue debt we couldn't pay.

Mark had other concerns as well. "Charlie isn't worried about where he's going to be at Christmas or whether anyone wants him," he said. "He's here. He's loved and taken care of, and that doesn't have to change. I don't feel compelled to make that official by adopting him."

When I spoke with the social worker and explained some of the reasons we hesitated with formally making Charlie our own child, she understood. But she had to deal with the protocol of planning for the permanency hearings, which required finding a home that would be considered the "adoptive resource." If we didn't choose to be that family, Charlie could be placed in another home. We'd had no luck finding someone qualified to care for all of Charlie's needs while Mark and I took a much-needed break. So finding an adoptive home for him seemed to be a stretch, but there was a slight possibility someone would be willing to adopt him.

I knew it was not in anyone's best interest for me to press the issue with my husband. It's difficult enough already to do foster care without having one partner say, "I never wanted to do this," and making the foundation insecure. In our marriage, we hardly have to have a good reason for Mark and me to annoy each other. My insisting on adopting if he didn't want to adopt would have been a recipe for disaster.

I prayed—and not some trite bullet "God bless this food, amen" kind of prayer either.

One poignant memory I have is of standing for worship at church. I couldn't find the breath to sing and understood Hannah's prayer to God for a child in ways I had not known before. The intensity of her prayers, rendering her unable to make a sound, gave the priest Eli the impression she was drunk, but oh, she was not. Fervently praying, yes. Inebriated, no.

My experience and prayer was similar: *God, I have no idea whether I'm going to be able to continue to take care of this child in the future. I'm not assuming I'm more capable or better than anyone else. I also am not presuming I personally have the strength and wherewithal to see it through until he dies. What I do know is that I want to be willing to do what You desire. If You are going to continue to provide for Charlie; if You know, because You've given me such a deep love for this baby, that any obstacles will be overcome, then here am I, Lord; pick me. I can do all things through Christ who strengthens me. And You work in Mark's heart. I will not attempt to convince him against his will that this is a good idea.*

I did not pray this prayer out loud. The evidence that I was having such an intense conversation, willing to give it all up or continue, was my silent tears. I remember using one of Charlie's clean cloth diapers to mop my face of the tears, the snot, and the mascara, because the tissue I had was failing to hold it all.

A couple of days later, Mark walked into the dining room where I was sitting and asked abruptly, "You really want to adopt that baby?"

"Yes."

"Then let's do it. Call the social worker. Get it going."

This was one of the most concise, yet monumental, discussions of our married life.

I called Faith right away, not out of fear Mark would change his mind, but because I believed God had directly answered my prayers and had moved in Mark's heart and mind to be in agreement.

The concerns over the van and house accommodations

were still niggling, but we pushed them aside. Every time I would have to lift Charlie and his wheelchair into the back of the van, I would pray, not even prefacing my prayer with God's name because He knew full well I was talking to Him every time I thought or said it: *I don't know how much longer I'll be able to lift him, but I'll have to do it for as long as it's necessary. You know I can feel impatient, even afraid of the possibility You might not provide, but You want me to trust You, so I'm going to act as if I do.*

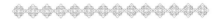

Most days, having a handicapped van seemed unnecessary because, honestly, our little buddy was not expected to live long enough to get so big he couldn't be managed.

As the next six months unfolded, Charlie would stop breathing adequately and his oxygen saturations would drop into dangerously low territory. We would go rushing about trying to remedy the situation, not altogether sure what was ailing him and causing the trouble in the first place. How could a child *on a ventilator* drop his sats out and turn gray? We didn't get an explanation for his breath-ing issues* until much later.

---

* trachea/bronchial malacia

When Charlie had his episodes, I had to work with the special needs on-call physician and troubleshoot the issue. The doctors and I would sift through the circumstances surrounding every breathing incident Charlie had with a nit comb. Questions went back and forth until the doctors figured out as much as humanly possible about why Charlie was having trouble. They pointed out what I had done effectively or ineffectively to deal with it. The scrutiny was not meant to be an inquisition even when I was at fault due to ignorance. I learned a lot in the first year Charlie was with us, and each time I would think it was too hard and too scary, but I had to wade back in because there was no quitting. I also learned something each time that helped me the next time he had a similar episode, making it less frightening to deal with. And then came the day when my best efforts appeared to be useless.

10

STRENGTH MADE PERFECT IN WEAKNESS

Jesus loves me—He will stay,
Close beside me all the way.
Then His little child will take,
Up to heaven for His dear sake.
Yes, Jesus loves me!
Yes, Jesus loves me!
Yes, Jesus loves me!
The Bible tells me so.

—Anna Bartlett Warner, "Jesus Loves Me"

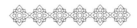

The first Saturday in October 2015, I had completed all the paperwork necessary to move forward with Charlie's adoption. It had been as intrusive a process as the foster care application. The questionnaire asks such personal questions as "Describe your first experience having sex."

Jaw dropping. You're kidding me, right?

I wrote, "I got married. We had sex. It was fine."

Good grief. I was not going to go into the fine points for people I knew, let alone people I did not know.

Questions were asked about how I felt about my childhood.

Let's see. I could go from happy to sad to tearful to mad to ecstatic to irritated—all in the space of an hour. Toss in a monthly period and I could have dramatic changes in how

I felt about life in general in the space of a minute.

I answered, "Happy."

Once more I was required to detail the events leading up to my night on the psych ward in December 2010. This go 'round I was very careful to fully explain what had happened so there wouldn't be any misperception about it. We had been thoroughly vetted before being able to be licensed as foster parents, but each and every time you want to move forward with an adoption, you get to go through the inquisition again. For those with only sweetness and light in their pasts, it would be a breeze. I have failed miserably in mine, and it threatens to define me every time my life is recounted and weighed in the balances, and I await the verdict on the human front.

On God's front, I know my standing. I am a sinner who has been saved by grace. I'm enough because God declares it so. This does not mean that my sinful choices are ignored and irrelevant when people are evaluating them. It simply means I'm complete in Christ.

I ran to the post office and mailed the packet of information. I sighed and thought there should be no glitches with Charlie's adoption, but I was prepared for the possibility that something unanticipated could pop up.

After I arrived home, I walked through the family room and did the once-over for Charlie, who was lying in bed. I checked the fluids in the humidifier, his feeding-tube pump, his oxygen saturation levels, the vent settings, his color, and his diaper, and I then proceeded to fine-tune from there.

I changed the bud's diaper, which was wet, and then turned him on his left side since he had been lying on his back for a while. We'd had him for almost a year, and what a ride it had been!

He didn't need to be suctioned, so my brain wasn't triggered to look at the suction machine.

This was a mistake.

I kissed his smoochable smooth cheek, stroked his head, and told him for the gazillioneth time, "I love you, baby boy!" Then I stepped about ten feet away through the doorway into the kitchen to get things prepared for lunch. I whirled around abruptly when Charlie's pulse oximeter alarmed, indicating he wasn't breathing properly. The alarm can go off if he wiggles the toe holding the probe too much, so I didn't immediately assume he was in trouble.

Oh, but he was.

That fast. Two minutes tops and he was already gray.

I flipped him onto his back and tried to suction his trach. The suction machine had gotten too full and hadn't been emptied. It wasn't working. His oxygen levels were in the low 80s by that point. The vent alarms were going off obnoxiously, the pulse ox was beeping loudly, signaling trouble. I raced across the room to the Go-bag to grab the portable suction machine and raced back to Charlie's bedside.

His saturations were now in the 70s.

Mary Elisabeth and Andrew came into the family room.

Andrew began to bounce back and forth on either side of the bed, trying to silence the alarms, but the problem was still there, so the quiet was only momentary. Mary Elisabeth asked what I needed, and I shouted, "Call 911!!"

She stood there.

She didn't want to do it. She didn't like *talking to people*. She peppered me with questions: "If Charlie is going to die, then why do I have to call 911 anyway? What am I supposed to tell them? Why do I even need to call? Why are you freaking out, Mom?"

I did *not* want to be having a conversation about Charlie's full code status and my duty. My understanding at the time was that I was his foster mom, not his real mom, and I had to do everything possible to make sure he continued to breathe and have a heart rate.

In spite of her not completely understanding why, Mary Elisabeth finally made the call and told the dispatcher to send help right away.

Andrew's bopping back and forth silencing the alarms to decrease some of the tension was driving me a little crazier. By this time my little boy's skin was dark gray and his lips purple, and his eyes were rolled back in his head, his body motionless. Needless to say, I was frantic.

I yelled at Charlie, "What? Do you think you're going to do this today? Today? I just put the adoption paperwork in the mail, for goodness' sake! Breathe!"

Unbeknownst to me, his lungs had filled with secretions when I turned him on his left side. He was drowning in his own fluids.

For me this was my nightmare of all nightmares, and it was happening right in front of me. It was horrible to watch and not be able to make the difference for him—the difference I had been helpless to make for my sister because I hadn't been there.

During those moments, Emily came through the doorway, asking what I wanted her to do. Oddly enough, I told her to clean up the kitchen! The look on her face told me I was nuts, but she did an about-face and walked back in to do as I asked.

Yeah, you read that correctly, I told my daughter to clean the kitchen.

When my life is in chaos, I have a tendency to straighten up messes in the house. If I'm able to restore order in some small fashion, I feel better able to deal with the parts I can't control.

At that point, Mark, having heard the rushing footfalls and hollering downstairs, came out of our room on the second floor, down the stairs, and burst onto the scene. I cried out feeling panicked, "It's not working! It's not working!"

Charlie's oxygen saturations had dropped to 30 percent, then nothing, at the same time his heart rate slowly dipped lower and then disappeared also.

Mark tilted Charlie's head back to open his airway while I worked to clear the fluid filling his lungs. My worst-case scenario was coming true. I was inadequate for the task, and this baby was going to die as a result.

Every family member present was praying in some fashion or another. The sirens coming down the street from the paramedics and fire department reached our ears.

I told Charlie one more time, wailing, "I don't want them to have to pound on your chest, baby. Please, please, breathe." I continued breathing efforts with the resuscitation air bag because it was my responsibility.

Ten minutes had passed since the first alarm had gone off. It was an eternity.

Suddenly Charlie gasped, then his chest moved and air flowed in.

I continued to bag him for another minute or two, and then Mark put the ventilator back in place once his oxygen saturation levels and heart rate began registering once more on the pulse oximeter.

There is no human reason Charlie began to breathe again. I'm fully convinced God was not ready to bring him home.

The EMS guys began streaming into the house from the front where Andrew had met them and was directing the traffic. A sea of blue uniforms and concerned faces surrounded us. As the men stepped close to the bed to get a good look at Charlie, Mark told them, "You know, guys, he's fine."

I snapped at Mark, clipping my words out tersely so no one could mistake how serious I was. "We are going to the hospital. He. Is. Not. Fine."

I was totally rattled and angry that my husband was treating the whole situation so lightly. Granted, it's his defense mechanism. He wants calm, and he'll pretend it exists if he needs to. I have been slow to learn that my going to even more extreme measures to help the man understand "it is not fine at all," are received with equal amounts of resistance.

The firemen and paramedics looked wary. I'm sure they wondered if they had a code blue on their hands or a domestic violence call. I left and went to the living room.

Shaken, I called our special needs liaison at Children's Hospital. Beth answered, and I told her what had just happened.

She was sympathetic and asked me to describe what Charlie looked like now.

I left the living room and walked back through the dining and kitchen area to where Charlie lay in the family room. He was breathing via the ventilator. His heart rate was normal for him, but he was unresponsive. He was lying so very still. He didn't react to the paramedic's attempts to elicit a pain response.

I choked on a sob and told Beth, "I'm not sure if he's brain-dead now. We have to come to Children's. I can't watch him myself and make that determination. And if he's brain-dead, we have a whole different scenario on our hands with this life-support business than we did if he's brain-damaged."

She agreed and told me she would make the phone calls necessary to have the ER ready to receive him when we arrived.

I pointedly ignored my husband, poor guy, and told the paramedics with a no-nonsense tone, "We are going to the hospital."

Rod, the supervisor of the EMS guys, nodded yes and got his men going to prepare for transport. Charlie was put on the cart and gently loaded into the back of the rig. The back doors shut, and the ambulance drove out of Sheboygan toward Milwaukee.

I looked down at my sweet boy, where he lay not moving. The only indication Charlie was still with us were his vital signs registering on the pulse ox. My thoughts were racing, and I was still attempting to tamp down the panic this child had created in my heart. I had fallen deeply in love with Charlie, so the potential hurt his death could cause was great. I was grieving but also trying not to lose it because it was not about me in that moment but about my child. He was the focus. I would have to find time later to fall apart.

We traveled mostly in silence. Rod was so gentle and kind in the way he handled Charlie. He gave me sympathetic glances, but this smart man seemed to know better than to ask how I was doing lest my facade of control slip and the dam of emotion break.

I held Charlie's right hand in mine, my thumb placed in the middle of his sweet palm with his fingers loosely wrapped around it. There was no clenching tightly of me to him, or him to me, or to life itself. He was unresponsive, and I was trying to hold loosely to his life, and his hand, because as Corrie ten Boom would say, "I must learn to hold earthly things lightly because, if I do not, the Lord might have to pry away my fingers, and that might hurt"[1] and "Never be afraid to trust an unknown future to a known God."[2]

We were nearly to the hospital, every possible scenario having passed through my mind, when Charlie spontaneously picked up his head and slowly turned it to the right side so he was facing me. He then extended his right arm toward my face, letting go of my thumb but pressing his hand out toward me. This was his signature way of asking for a kiss. I held his hand in mine and immediately pressed my lips to his sweet palm where my thumb had been.

I caught myself tearing up and murmured, "Oh buddy, you're back. You're back."

By the time we got into the ER and he was evaluated, the medical staff asked me, "How does he look to you right now?" Charlie can be scary to the casual observer with the way his eyes don't focus, but I told them with a rueful laugh, "He looks like a million bucks. But he sure didn't two hours ago. I know I have to take him home. He can't live here, but I want you to know it is terrifying to be helpless when he's drowning in his secretions like that."

I turned away so overcome I couldn't continue. I ducked into the bathroom, gently closing the door, and slid down the wall, quietly sobbing, unable to hold in my emotions any longer. I whispered through the cascade of tears raining down my cheeks, "Dear God, wasn't it enough to have him be medically fragile, not terminal? And then needing a ventilator? And then I'm responsible for keeping him alive at all costs, and now he could drown right in front of me? I'm not sure I'm able to do this. I thought we had some ground rules? I told You what I wanted, what kind of good I hoped to effect in his life, and the very thing that was horrible about Amie's death is a reality." And while gulping air, my chest heaving, I wailed, "And Charlie's not ever even going to go swimming!"

My heart was breaking over this cross I had been asked to carry.

When I finally pulled myself together and emerged from the bathroom, the doctor saw I was back at Charlie's bedside, and he returned and said compassionately, "I'm not sending you home today. We're going to see if there is something we can do to figure out why he stops breathing even while being ventilated. Hang in there with me a couple of days."

Sunday morning as I sat on the couch across the room from Charlie, I kept my distance. I was afraid of the power this child had to scare me half out of my mind. I wasn't consciously putting space between us; but physically, in that small room, we couldn't be any farther apart. The nurse asked me a couple of times if I wanted her to get him settled on my lap. I answered, "We'll wait a little while. Thanks."

She inquired again a few hours later, pressing for a firmer time.

"Uh, well, the Packers game is on this afternoon. Maybe then," I said.

The nurse did not let me get away with putting it off any longer but came in before the game started, and with a matter-of-fact attitude, she said, "Let's get you set up. I'm going to lunch, and want to have Charlie situated before I do."

I sat in the recliner next to my buddy's bed. She picked him up, placed him in my lap, arranged all the wires and tubing attached to his body, and left us to ourselves.

I looked down at the precious child lying in my arms and realized again, *There is a baby underneath all this equipment. Don't ever forget that, Salchert.*

I found out that the old idiom "If you fall off a horse, the best thing to do is get back on as soon as possible" was true.

My fear that Charlie would die was real, and it was also greater than my love as long as he was not close to me. Putting that baby in my arms was the best way God could help me draw close to him again. While I still felt fear, it wasn't the reigning emotion or driving force anymore. Something greater was at stake, and Charlie was worth every tear I would shed or any fear I would face in caring for him.

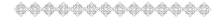

We spent about four days in the hospital. The doctors ordered all kinds of tests to be run on Charlie to determine, if possible, why it was he could stop breathing effectively even while on a ventilator.

I was able to stay at the Ronald McDonald House.

One evening I was very thankful there was no one in the kitchen while I was preparing my supper. I was peopled out, just plain tired of interacting, and I wanted to be alone, but I couldn't eat in my room because that was against the house rules.

I had finished my meal and was cleaning up when a man came up the stairs and pulled a plate and fork out of the cupboard and drawer. He headed to the main dining area to get the meal some wonderfully benevolent group had prepared.

I stood by the sink, madly scrubbing the pans I had used, thinking, *Hurry up, sister, or he'll be back and you'll have to* talk *to him!*

I was too slow in spite of my best efforts.

He came back and sat at the counter, his shoulders hunched, his dejected demeanor evoking sympathy on my part even though I was exhausted.

I asked my usual question of others who stay at Ronald McDonald House: "What're ya in for?"

He told me his seventeen-year-old was at a critical point. The doctors had told him if she didn't respond to treatment in the next day or two, they weren't sure she would make it.

Oh, my heart ached for his grief and pain, and I could empathize not just sympathize.

We were both Christians and quickly discovered our commonality and then could more deeply encourage each other to hang in there. Rehearsing our different histories of the way God was in the business of answering prayers left us both much more optimistic, hopeful, and inspired at the end of the conversation. Exactly what the doctor would have ordered! Ha!

A couple of days later, while I was getting lunch, I saw him and his daughter. I hugged the man then I hugged his daughter and exclaimed, "My goodness, you're out of the hospital!"

"Yes! We got our miracle! She got out on a special pass

just to have a lunch together, and then she is going to be discharged soon and come home more permanently."

What a fantastic answer to heartfelt prayers. I was so happy for them!

Our situation received answers to prayer, too, but not so dramatically. Charlie's test results did not reveal anything helpful.

During Thursday morning rounds, I stood in the doorway of Charlie's room and faced the attending physician, a number of resident doctors, his nurse, and the case manager.

"There's nothing left to do for him medically, is there?" I questioned.

Shaking their heads no, shifting back and forth on their feet, all the personnel present obviously badly wanted to tell me something could be fixed and we could go home hopeful and relieved.

I looked at the attending doctor, who had been especially kind, patient, and understanding of my fears and Charlie's prognosis, and said, "It's okay. We do have answers because we know what can't be fixed now. We're going to go home. We are going to live like we're going to be here another hundred years, but we're also going to live like today is our last day with this baby boy. I am full of hope, just not in any kind of medical procedure. You've done all you can do, and we're grateful. I'm ready to take him home, and we won't necessarily need to come back. Thank you for everything, honestly, thank you."

There was no way to stop Charlie from having the episodes where he couldn't breathe because his airways collapsed or filled with fluid. We would go home and deal with his day-to-day fragility. My hospice background is a gift. I am able to shift focus from finding a cure to making the very best of a tough, incurable situation. It was awful to hear that he would continue to have trouble until he ultimately died from it, but it was a relief to know we had exhausted our options and weren't missing some vital piece of information.

Our palliative care doctor, Dr. Jack, was a godsend during those days I wrestled with the reality that Charlie wasn't going to be with us on my initial terms. If I didn't want to deal with the possibility of his drowning, then I would effectively be saying I didn't want him. This grievous conclusion was not a viable option. Someone had to stay close to this baby when he died, someone who knew him and could be a comfort because of familiarity. I did not want him dying alone or surrounded by strangers. I worked through my options where his care was concerned, and Jack listened carefully and gave tangible solutions when possible. Medications, such as morphine and Ativan, could be prescribed, which help with air hunger and the panic that ensues when Charlie can't get his breath. The meds would also allow Charlie's airways to relax so breathing interventions might be more effective.

Charity, Mary Elisabeth, Andrew, and Emily came to the hospital and attended a meeting I had arranged with Dr. Jack especially for them. I knew the events of the Saturday before had left us all more than a little upset. I wasn't assuming my children understood what had happened since then, so Dr. Jack asked them if they wanted out and would prefer to leave Charlie in the hospital.

They went around the room and said things like, "No, he can come home. We just don't get why 911 had to be called, because if he's going to die, why are we calling them to come? Emmalynn's death was so calm and peaceful.

When mom is freaking out, we feel like freaking out, so she can't be doing that anymore!" (All of my children there echoed this sentiment.) Their questions were answered fairly satisfactorily; sometimes the answer was "I don't know." And while they definitely were given the choice not to invite Charlie home again, none of them opined that he should stay at the hospital.

They weighed in and told us, "Charlie's death needs to be clean, not a secret we're ashamed of. We need to be able to talk about it, how he died, not just when. We need to know he wasn't suffering because of us. We need to know we were with him, gave him medications at the prescribed dose, and were available to try to clear his airway of whatever was blocking it."

Our family also understands that because of a 2002 Wisconsin legal case ruling, *Montalvo v. Borkovec*, Charlie cannot truly be a hospice patient. The Wisconsin State legislature says, "In the absence of a persistent vegetative state, the right of a parent to withhold life-sustaining treatment from a child does not exist."[3]

Charlie is not in a persistent vegetative state. Charlie doesn't have a lethal anomaly. Charlie doesn't necessarily have a terminal diagnosis. So, by law in Wisconsin, we are required to pound on his chest and call 911 and have paramedics do compressions and defibrillation plus administer medications to get his heart restarted.

Charlie experiences apnea, flaccid airways,* and nonepileptic seizure activity when he is in pain. The very activity of resuscitation would be yet another reason he wouldn't survive the efforts. A "code" is always painful, though it is not always successful.

*tracheobrochomalacia

We are such public figures now that we have been told we could be sued by those who might feel we were negligent in not using full code measures on Charlie. We can't go back and become just another family on Third Street. But it's an undue burden for our family to have legislation dictating the extent we must go to bring Charlie back should he have an episode of central/obstructive apnea and his heart stop as a result. I don't even know what kind of help we need for it to be legal for us to allow Charlie to die as naturally as possible. This is the burden we have been asked to bear on Charlie's behalf. And sometimes there are no words to describe how heavy it is. Like the example Jesus set of "for the *joy* set before him he endured the cross" (Hebrews 12:2 NIV, emphasis added), all this pain and heartache will be worth it.

I take the tenth chapter of Hebrews to heart. Verse 39 is one of my favorites: "But we're not quitters who lose out. Oh, no! We'll stay with it and survive, trusting all the way" (MSG).

11

CRAZY AMAZING
ANSWERS TO PRAYER

He comes "to bind the brokenhearted";
He comes the fainting soul to cheer;
He gives me "oil of joy" for mourning,
And "beauty for ashes" here.

—John G. Crabbe, "Beauty for Ashes"

After Charlie was discharged from the hospital, I was relieved of the necessity of chasing any and all possibilities of improving his health. We had pretty much run out of curative options. I prayed and asked God to redeem and help heal the sadness I felt over coming to terms with our focus shifting to palliative care.

Our family had come to appreciate the paramedics and firemen who had raced to our home to help us time and again during the past year. I was then struck by the fact that we had called our local EMS more than twenty times through the years. They had responded, done a wonderful service, and the most I had done for them was bellyache over the bill I received in the mail.

What a sad commentary.

I was determined this would change. The men and women both deserved and should be shown our gratitude for their selfless service on our behalf. So we made twenty dozen oatmeal-raisin cookies and invited both the Orange

Cross and the Sheboygan Fire Department to our home to have the treats and take a large tray of them back to the station for those who couldn't come. Most importantly, this allowed us to personally say a huge thank-you for all they had done.

Both emergency services departments were more than happy to accommodate our request. They don't always get to go to people's homes for nonemergency reasons. This was a sweet reason to show up at our door. The Sheboygan Fire Department was so moved by our gesture that they asked us to bring Charlie to the fire station, which was ten blocks away and housed the ambulance crew who most frequently responded to our calls. About fifteen of the guys gathered, and these kind men made Charlie an official honorary firefighter with a brief ceremony. They gave him a fleece blanket with a fire-engine pattern and tied edges. They also gave him a onesie with the company logo. Making him their "little brother" was a heartfelt gift on their part. They have continued with this allegiance to him even though they have had to transport him only a couple of times in the two years following his near-fatal coding.

Our foster care agency was touched by the way our hometown heroes reached out and embraced Charlie. Foster kids want to feel as if they belong and are part of the community, putting down roots in the home or city where they live.

The public relations department at Children's Hospital in Milwaukee reached out after Charlie's adoption, or "Gotcha Day," on December 18, 2015, and asked if we would be willing to do a media release about foster care and adoption. We agreed.

Leah Ulatowski, a reporter from the *Sheboygan Press*, came to our home armed with a notebook and a cell phone. She sat with me and Charlie, asking question after question. I asked her a couple of times if we were done, wanting to be courteous with her time. She assured me we were good. Her compassion and interest were real.

Leah went back to the office and crafted a beautiful article. The website version was released on Saturday, January 2, 2016, and the *Sheboygan Press* ran it on Sunday's front page. All of a sudden, the story went viral. Who would've thunk it?

Oh wait. . . . God knew!

We had not anticipated anyone in Sheboygan would read about our baby boy, let alone have our story go worldwide. One of the people who saw the article was Terri Peters at *TODAY*. Terri was willing to let me further explain why we do what we do. She gathered material from me via email, edited it, and presented the story as an as-told-to segment in June 2016. This story went viral too.

Soon after a literary agent asked if I would like to write a book.

"I can't *not* write" was one of the things I said. As much as I would like to shut up and not say anything, Ravi Zacharias affirms my desire to chronicle our journey:

> "This pause to remember is indispensable in our sacred memory. Only as we remember and remind ourselves of God's faithfulness can we even see the pattern God has woven in our lives and learn confidence in His working. That is why, on repeated occasions, God tells the people to place a stone or a marker to remind them to tell the next generation of what God had done."[1]

People, *Reader's Digest*, *Guideposts*, and numerous other publications printed various versions of our story. When *People* asked to interview our family in February 2016 to document a day in the life of Charlie, my response had more than a little, "You're kidding me, right?" attitude when I told her, "A day in the life of Charlie? Okay, hold on to your hat—it's riveting material. We change his diaper; we lotion his skin. We suction his mouth and trach. We turn on the CD player so he can jam to the Gaithers or Joey Feek, and we do the same things pretty much over and over again. Toss in a bath and a dance or two in the kitchen, and that's our buddy's life."

After getting off the phone with the reporter, I seriously contemplated not having them come at all. It seemed ludicrous. But God provided perspective.

Mark and I had inquired a few weeks previously about a baby boy named Samuel whose foster care bio asked for a family, not even one to take him home, but someone willing to come sit by his bedside so he wasn't always alone. He was a couple of months older than Charlie and hadn't ever been able to leave the hospital. This was not the only kind of life he could have. We had evidence of that fact in our own family room!

Before we could even get any traction to move Samuel home with us, I received this email:

> *With my deepest regrets I have to inform you the child you inquired about, Samuel, passed away yesterday. I want to personally thank you for opening your hearts and potentially your home.*

The social worker included the obituary published in the paper.

The little angel Samuel, Born 11/24/2013—Passed from this earth on 2/9/2016.

> Samuel was a permanent-custody child. He was in foster care his entire life and had always been in the hospital since his birth. Due to the circumstances under which he was born, Samuel was unable to sustain any meaningful quality of life. He is now at peace without the pain and suffering he endured while on earth. He now has the eternal quality of life he deserves and is rejoicing with the angels in heaven.

"No meaningful quality" would not be the summation of Charlie's life. And that helped me to realize that *People* most assuredly should come and let the world know the difference a family's love and a whole lot of smooching and hand holding could make.

Charlie's life has touched millions of people. Millions. He has had an impact on them in ways we never could have fathomed. One mom contacted me via Facebook and told me that she and her husband had lost a daughter who was only twelve. They had been foster parents, but after their own biological child died, they could not deal with the grief of having to say good-bye to another kiddo, even if it was so that child could be placed back with their birth parents. This couple had been hurt and couldn't fathom asking for more heartache on purpose. She told me that they decided that if our family could willingly take on this kind of burden with children who were pretty much guaranteed a shortened life, then they could be braver than they thought possible too.

A few weeks later she sent me another note with this excited message:

We did it. Called our social worker and told him we wanted back in the game. We hardly had to wait any time before we were given a little girl in a wheelchair that had been difficult to place. She's home with us now. Thank you for the push to get us going again!

Countless others have reached out to me to share stories of their children who have varying disabilities. The isolation they have felt isn't so great after having been able to commiserate and be cheered on, emboldened to speak up on behalf of their child, and empowered to fight for what is needed enthusiastically and a little less fearfully.

One of my favorite quotes is "We read to know we are not alone."[2] I firmly believe that. Reading about Charlie and Emmalynn and our mind-set in caring for the least of these helps others step up and boldly do it too.

What I know for sure is that if God disabled me physically because He desired for me to be at home with the children He had already given me and with any other baby He might bring along my path, I am willing to be faithful there. He had crushed me to remove the self-seeking desires I'd had to do things my own way. Running on up ahead of Him or lagging behind, unwilling to follow cheerfully, had caused me so much trouble. I had endured great heartache trying to do things my way.

I cringe when I hear people brag about how amazing and invincible they are, or when they brag about their physical or mental abilities. In a breath it can all be gone. Consider all the football players who brag about how great they are, only to be seen standing on the sidelines wearing a ball cap and sweats because an injury took them out and revealed they were human and breakable too.

I found this out about myself. God broke my heart, my spirit, and my body. And I'm grateful. I don't need a job or relationships or any children or material things to make me feel valuable.

He calls me His own.

I'm safe with Him.

I'm accepted.

I'm not too much.

I'm not too little.

I'm not perfect and not expected to be. I'm under construction, and God is working all things together for good because He loves me. I have experienced the shattering He has brought about, not to destroy me, but to make me into the kind of woman who radiates the love of her Savior. Everything in this life I might want to hold on to may be taken in an instant. God had to take mostly everything away in order for me to be able to receive it back in the way He intended.

A portion of the poem "Treasures" explains how I felt:

One by one He took them from me,
All the things I valued most.
Until I was empty-handed,
Every glittering toy was lost. . . .
Then at last I comprehended,
With my stupid mind and dull,
That God could not pour out His riches,
Into hands already full.[3]

I find it telling that near the end of *Rosemary: The Hidden Kennedy Daughter*, this is included:

> "The interest [Rosemary] sparked in my family towards people with special needs," Anthony [Kennedy Shriver] claims, "will one day go down as the greatest accomplishment that any Kennedy has made on a global basis. . . ."
>
> [Eunice Kennedy Shriver], however, would be the most powerful moving force behind the cause of the disabled, pushing public and private institutions and foundations to sponsor and provide services, to fund and conduct research, and to make accommodations for the intellectually and physically challenged. Once locked away or institutionalized, people with developmental, intellectual, psychological, and physical disabilities can now participate in life and integrate in communities in ways that seemed impossible when Rosemary was a child and young adult."[4]

This is my story—of the redemption (and it's not even all done yet!) of my beloved sister Amie's life and tragic death! It is one I have been privileged to share repeatedly with numerous doctors, nurses, therapists, reporters and photographers, churches, and EMS personnel. If folks are only looking at me, they will be disappointed because I'm a deeply flawed human being.

But if they happen to be looking at me and are paying attention, then God willing, what they will see and hear is my making much of a great God who saved a wretch like me and is effecting good in the lives He brings across my path. Not for my glory but for His.

June 2016, a year from the time God answered my Hannah-like prayer and Mark gave me the go-ahead to adopt, I made an appointment for Charlie to get a second opinion from a neurologist. I wasn't sure whether Charlie's brain had continued to deteriorate and fill up with cerebrospinal fluid or if it was holding steady. Was he going to die or not?

I know what a person looks like who is actively dying, and Charlie wasn't exhibiting any of those signs or symptoms. However, he certainly flirted with death at any given time related to the malacia. Dr. E ordered a new MRI of Charlie's brain and compared it to the one taken the previous year.

He told me what he thought, and then he also showed me the differences in the MRIs and shared his opinion on Charlie's prognosis: "Your baby is obviously well taken care of. You attend to him quickly and expertly. He's thriving in spite of his condition. I saw you playing with him, enjoying him. You love him. Period. This child may die at any time because his tracheostomy could obstruct, but you need to also understand, given the level of care he receives, you could also be looking at another ten to twelve years before he'll be actively dying. At that point his brain will not be able to keep up with the neurological demands his body will place on it."

I left the office in Green Bay with Charity and Charlie in tow, and we drove home. I felt a little shell-shocked. I had thought Charlie was going to die sooner than later, but I was certainly not wishing he would. I was confused and felt a little stupid. For the nearly two years he had needed assistance to clear his airway and bagging to help restore his oxygen levels, I had assumed something was giving out that would result in death. Thinking that he could be doing this for another ten to twelve years was disconcerting.

I was fifty years old, and Mark was sixty-one at the time. We were looking at a longer timeline of caring for this child, years longer than we had anticipated. The weight of it rolled over me like a tank.

There was no "I quit. Give him back. I didn't sign up for this." It was more a matter of, How in the world were we going to be able to care for this baby as he grew in length and got heavier and more difficult to physically manage? One of the biggest obstacles was the expense of a van equipped to handle his wheelchair with him in it. He is one with his chair. A twenty-pound ventilator is mounted on the side. Our van did not have working air conditioning. Now, my usual thought is *Don't whine. Roll the windows down and drive fast and just suck it up, buttercup.*

But Charlie cannot handle extreme heat or cold.

We did not have the money to buy a wheelchair-accessible van. It was something we had talked about but felt as if it were a moot point with Charlie's medical condition being so fragile. When we signed up to adopt him, we didn't feel as though we were out of our financial league, because he was not expected to live long enough for a van to be an issue.

God has a beautiful sense of humor. He absolutely wanted Charlie adopted and set that lonely boy in our family by His design. He also knew our hesitation about agreeing to something that we could not foreseeably afford.

As noted earlier, when Mark and I got married, we had sex. Our eldest daughter popped out in February 1989, nine months and four hours after our wedding day. We didn't have two nickels to rub together, but each of us, separate from each other, came to the same conclusion and felt convicted that we didn't know squat about figuring out the timing of having children. If we were trusting God with our eternal souls, then in our opinion, we would be just fine trusting Him with the provision of the children He gave us.

I write that now, seeing how peculiar it was to be convinced God would provide for the children He enabled us to conceive but doubting whether He would provide for a child we adopted. How hilariously silly to think otherwise.

As I have read through the Old Testament, over and over I have seen the phrase, "And this has happened so you may know that I am the LORD your God." Trials, suffering, blessing, fertility, success, failure—everything was brought about so that the people God was dealing with would know He was the Lord. When I read this, my perspective changed, and now I fully understand that God is unchanging. We have biblical accounts of how God has worked to show us that we are not alone, uniquely experiencing random and meaningless trials.

In a conversation with our Palliative Care doctor, I told him, whispering because I couldn't say it any louder because of the tears, "You know, even knowing what I know now about how difficult it's going to be to keep Charlie, I still would have suited up and played the game."

Dr. Jack nodded both in agreement and confidence, "Yes. You would have."

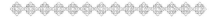

One story of how God met our ongoing needs in a miraculous way came about through the most unlikely circumstances.

The event coordinator for Keller Williams Realty contacted me in October 2016 and invited me to the realty's annual training event called the Family Reunion. She said that vice chairman Mo Anderson had read an article about Charlie. Mo was so emotionally moved that she insisted I come to the event.

This baffled me. We don't have a Keller Williams agency in Sheboygan; I had never even seen the red KW logo. My home was not for sale, and I was not looking for a home, so I had no idea why my presence was requested. My sweet girlfriend Bonnie, who helps manage my email accounts, told me I should absolutely follow up on this. KW is quite a large organization, and she had a hunch it would be important for me to say yes.

I contacted KW and said I was willing to go to Vegas in February. I chatted with Mo and three other Keller Williams employees in a conference call. They asked me what our family needed to take care of Charlie. This question usually leaves me a little stumped. My philosophy when it comes to stuff is "less is better." I don't want cleaning my house to take a long time, so I keep clutter at a minimum. I told the ladies, "Diapers. Diapers are good."

"Yes, but what else might you need?" they persisted.

I hesitated; then, because they were waiting, I blurted: "A van. We need a van. Hauling Charlie's wheelchair with him in it and all his paraphernalia is getting tougher in the accommodations we have right now. I am not physically capable of carrying much more weight." I apologized and said hurriedly, "You asked. I told you. I'm sorry."

They instantly reassured me they were glad I had shared. The phone call ended right after that. I was dismayed. I sent an email immediately after our conversation to assure them my hand was not out. Mark and I take these kiddos and know God will provide for them. We weren't going around trying to drum up support or have people feel sorry for us, or even worse, using them for our own gain.

They wrote back and told me they were just fine. They didn't think I was asking for a handout, but they did encourage me to set up a Go-Fund Me account so we would be ready if the realtors who heard my story would want to contribute to a van fund.

I reviewed the script prepared by Mo's assistant, which amounted to about ten minutes of actual conversation. I debated in my heart if I should even go to Vegas. Geez Louise, KW was going to an awful lot of trouble to fly me out and pay for my hotel just to chat with Mo for a few minutes.

In the meantime Mark and I had been in the process of becoming foster parents to a terminally ill teenager we nicknamed T-bear. We had no idea if he would ever be stable enough to leave the hospital and come home.

A few weeks before the event, I was talking with my girls in the dining room. I told them I was heading to Vegas for a realtor's conference.

Their confusion was reflected on their faces. "You're not a realtor. Why would you go?"

"Well"—I hemmed and hawed and shrugged my shoulders sheepishly—"there's this inspirational morning. . ."

"Yeah, so? But why would *you* go?"

I laughed and adapted one of our favorite lines from the 1995 movie *Sabrina*: "Nobody is as inspirational as me, not even me!"[5]

Speaking in front of eighteen thousand people wasn't a source of concern for me. However, when I arrived and found out I was one of three people asked to be on stage with Mo the next day, I was momentarily flustered. The other two were amazing. I was "just a mom." I wasn't saving the world like this young girl who makes beautiful bags and stocks them with goodies for homeless women. I wasn't this charismatic lady who is renewing neighborhoods in Detroit and doing so in an effort to be the one to bring the change she wants to see. Shoot. I was casting about in my mind trying to find where I fit in. I finally gave a little resigned sigh and weakly reassured myself with the thought, *They asked me to come. I didn't ask them to be here. There must be something they believed was important enough to pick me.*

The day before the event, Mo reminded me to stick closely to the script because it helped her to know when to ask questions. She said, "When I ask you what you need for the children you care for, I want you to say, 'Diapers and a van.' Period. You don't have to explain. My people are smart and will know why. I have thousands of people in this audience who are generous and motivated givers. We are not going to share this story without giving them the ability to have action points."

When the morning arrived, I was the second inspirational story to be shared. For the life of me, I couldn't follow the prompts on the screen. My gut and ability to read were a little out of conscious control. (Silly of me to have thought I wouldn't be nervous.) I answered Mo's questions off the cuff, sharing my heart for these children, and I'm sure that threw her for a loop. The last question Mo asked me was about what we needed.

I shrugged my shoulders, shifting my weight around apologetically on the stool I was sitting on and said, "Diapers and a van," and proceeded to go into detail why. Out of the corner of my eye, I noticed Mo cough, so I abruptly shut up. She reached over and handed me a card, saying, "Well, here's a gift card for diapers," to which I responded, "Awesome."

And then she smiled and slyly looked out at the audience of her beloved Keller Williams Realty family, reached down to pick up my left hand with her right hand, and held it while simultaneously pressing a key against my palm and saying, "And here's the key to your new van!"

The audience instantly jumped to its feet, clapping and cheering.

I put my head down and wept.

I didn't have to hope I had been eloquent enough to move folks' hearts that morning. I wasn't in a competition with the other two ladies who were sharing their stories, to have the folks in the audience decide who should benefit from their generosity once the conference was over. It was no longer about being enough on any level. Relief flooded over me.

Leaving the conference, I met dozens of KW realtors at the airport, and they blew me away with their hugs and encouragement and kind responses to what I had shared that morning.

I came home thinking the van was a done deal. It was with a little confusion I realized it wasn't. It was wholly because God had more folks who needed to be touched and involved.

A minivan had been picked out sometime in the late fall of 2016, and at that point in time, we only had Charlie. The person who selected the van on our behalf didn't understand that Charlie not only traveled with his wheelchair but also had to remain in it. The chosen minivan could certainly have a wheelchair stored in the back but would not be able to handle Charlie sitting in it. We also had a new child in a wheelchair who needed to be transported.

The paperwork was delayed because so many people were involved in the interstate purchase. My husband and I were praying and came to the conclusion that we were grateful KW had been so gracious in bringing me out to Vegas to share Charlie's story on their dime, but the minivan in process of being acquired was not going to meet our needs. In our estimation the realtors who contributed to the KW Cares fund from their commissions worked hard for their money. I wanted to have integrity with the way it was spent, and if the van proposed was bought and then sold, and we couldn't afford another one that worked for us, and Charlie didn't benefit, the sacrifice was lost. We weren't in any way seeking to profit from having adopted Charlie or sharing our lives with the world. We had no desire to pocket more than $20,000 and then not use it for its intended purpose.

Plus we knew we were in the process of bringing T-bear into our home, and we would need a much larger van to fit two wheelchair-dependent boys. It wasn't Keller Williams's responsibility to keep flexing with our needs as the number of our children in wheelchairs fluctuated.

We fully gave up the right to have the original van promised and were content to wait until God met our exact needs, because He was the one who had made it possible for us to add another child to the mix. Astonishingly, I received an email from our KW contact asking if it would be all right for KW to give us a check for $25,000 so that we could buy a van ourselves that was appropriate for our family. We answered yes, and this was met with an enthusiastic, "Amazing! We'll get back to you soon."

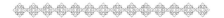

In March plans were being finalized to bring T-bear home. The day he arrived, Mark and I sat down with Make-A-Wish Foundation representatives for the second time to talk about Charlie's wish. Initially we had desired to take Charlie to the ocean in June for his third birthday in an RV in order to handle all of the equipment he uses. These plans were not formalized but rather had been put on hold as we were encouraged to give more thought to how we wanted to make that happen.

During that time frame, T-bear came along and into our care. I met with some of his physicians and mentioned our desire for the trip to the Pacific Ocean with Charlie, which would have occurred after T-bear was home with us.

This idea was met with a shaking of the head. T-bear was too medically fragile to travel far from the hospital. Expecting that he could handle a trip was totally unreasonable, and purposely putting him back in the hospital for two weeks while we made the journey with Charlie was not an option.

We shared with our Make-A-Wish representatives our reconciliation with not being able to go to the Pacific coast and our compelling desire to care for T-bear anyway, even if it caused us to give up the dream of getting to the ocean.

The ladies then asked about whether we had gotten a van yet that was equipped to handle both of their chairs. The answer was no, and I honestly had no idea when any of it was going to be resolved. They wanted us to consider the benefit of enhancing Charlie's life day to day by being able to ride in a van that was wheelchair accessible. We shared how he loves to take a drive to Lake Michigan, to

Grandma's house, and other places besides just the hospital or doctors' offices. His heart rate stabilizes and his eyes are open, looking all around. The windows are down whenever the weather permits, and the breeze blows his wispy hair. Riding in a van is something he really appears to enjoy.

Make-A-Wish had granted other people's requests for a van-accessorizing package. They would not provide the vehicle but could possibly accessorize one we already had. We had to be cautious in our expectations. Mark and I had no way of purchasing a van on our own, and the whole thing—both the Make-A-Wish Foundation's offer and KW's gift—might not materialize.

I felt a little foolish not having our ducks in a row. If I'm transparent, I have to say we have almost *never* had all our ducks in a row. Rather, we have squirrels that cannot be managed or controlled in any semblance of order. I prefer not to live this way. I like to know how everything is going to work out, and then I'll jump in and be crazy spontaneous. And God laughs and laughs. He, of course, knows the beginning from the end. I do not, and faith is what pleases Him, so He gives me tons of opportunities to throw up my hands and say, "I dunno how this is going to all work out, but You do, so do Your thing!"

Well, He did it in early April. Keller Williams sent a confirmation email that the check was in the mail. I had also heard from Make-A-Wish that our palliative care doctor had signed his approval of Charlie's wish to have a van makeover. I made contact with Make-A-Wish and told them we had the money to buy the van. At one point there seemed to be many loose ends, then suddenly all things were working together for our good.

I was driving home one day and saw a couple of Ford

Transit vans in the local Ford dealer's lot. I pulled in and walked around them and, to my delight, discovered the price tag on the one that would work best for our family was $22,999.

A sweet saleswoman helped me figure out the best way to move forward, the finance guy agreed on the price, a wheel-and-tire roadside assistance package was tossed in, and the total came to $25,004.45. Wildly enough, it was the exact van we were hoping to get; only because it was a year old and now a used vehicle, the price was almost $20,000 less. My frugal zealot's heart was singing!

I want to be generous to a fault, but I also dislike buyer's remorse because I have paid more than I should have. I signed the paperwork to put the van on hold while we waited for the check from KW to make it official.

A week later I was contacted by Make-A-Wish, and the representative told me that Charlie's Wish would come before the committee the next morning.

The next morning? Oh my. I kinda, sorta already thought it was settled. *Gulp.*

I never would have spent the entire 25 thousand on a newer van if I had known we might have to equip it too. Equipping a van comes with a hefty price tag, and I could not assume Charlie was more deserving or special than any other child asking for a dream to be fulfilled.

I woke up the next morning, and my heartfelt, simple prayer was a firm confidence in asking for my requests to be answered the way I wanted, but also holding on to the fact that my desires might not be what was best.

After missing a phone call and consciously choosing not to fret, I got a second call. The Make-A-Wish representative told me that, yes, we were granted the van accessory kit. She said she had actually cried at the meeting because she was so happy on our behalf.

Three months, not a week, after being told we were going to get a wheelchair-accessible van, the van was granted. It holds eight people in seats and a couple of wheelchairs in the back, fully equipped to meet the needs God knew our growing family would have.

God's eye is on the sparrow, and I *know* He watches me and provides over and abundantly above all we could ask or think (Ephesians 3:20).

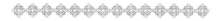

But wait, there's more! In May 2017 construction began on our home.

Mr. C, a generous and benevolent man, approached me and asked what would be helpful for our family to keep doing what we're doing. He asked me what I would need for a hospice room.

"A dresser and a bed" was my reply. No fancy stuff is necessary to care for these kiddos.

He pressed for more than that in regard to Charlie.

I was able to share a deep longing I had for a sunroom that could be used year-round. Winters in Wisconsin are long, and for at least six months out of the year, Charlie isn't able to be outside because he can't handle the near-freezing and subzero Wisconsin temperatures. He loves to be in the sunlight in our family room and often turns his face toward the light coming in through the window nearest his bed.

I shared with Mr. C and his friends and "cohorts in crime" that I had a longing for a beautiful sunroom so that those who were needed to be with Charlie would be excited about the opportunity and not reluctant to have to spend hours at his bedside attending to his needs. The group of men and women took it from there and designed a gorgeous space with five skylights so Charlie and companions can see the sun, sky, and clouds, and at night, the stars. Windows on all sides let in as much light as possible.

A wheelchair ramp has been built on the back of our home and a wheelchair-accessible shower installed in our main-floor bathroom. We are set up and ready to do this thing God has given us to do, without it being the physical challenge it was for a couple of years. I have learned to trust God every single day. We want what He wants and nothing less, even though it's seriously scary at times to ask Him to have His way, nothing held back.

Our lives are not magical. We are not lucky. We don't twitch our noses like a character on the TV show *Bewitched* and presto, things happen.

Time and again, the resolution to our prayers is multifaceted. It usually doesn't happen in the time frame I personally might allot for the answer to come; some of my prayer requests have taken forty years to be answered! Waiting doesn't discourage me as easily anymore but instead gives me courage to hold steady. God is working all things together for good. Even more typically, God works in mysterious ways, and more people are involved in the process than I could imagine.

12

STAINED GLASS WINDOWS

This is my story, this is my song,
Praising my Savior all the day long.

—FANNY JANE CROSBY, "BLESSED ASSURANCE"

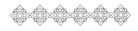

Taking care of and loving the children we have is a gift on many fronts. I regularly get opportunities to work out my faith and make it real. Day in and day out, Mark and I especially have to trade off leaving home. I run errands while he stays with the children we have at home, and then I come back and he goes. Lying on a beach or playing rounds of golf in Florida are just dreams, even though my husband, for sure, is old enough to retire, kick back, and take it easy.

We believe we're engaged in a good work that is pleasing to God. We are part of a team. Our biological kids help to care for the children we take into our home. We are in contact frequently with social workers, nurses, therapists, doctors, pharmacists, and other health-care professionals. Our team isn't accomplishing a sprint together but rather a marathon!

I have read numerous books by people who have suffered greatly and yet have come out on the other side better not bitter. Maybe not physically strong but stronger in spirit, not simply a shadow of themselves. My favorite kinds of movies involve individuals or teams who endure great adversity and overcome. I want to be one of those people.

As I worked on this book over the past year, time and again God met me on the page. There is not space enough to share all the ways He has redeemed the losses I have experienced as I have continually laid my hurt and pain before Him and asked Him in faith to redeem my losses, believing He would. He has never left me alone but has been with me and involved every step of the way.

Since reading the section "God Planned My Dad's Death" by Steve Saint in the book *Suffering and the Sovereignty of God*, I have considered his words and taken them to heart. He writes about the spearing deaths of five missionaries who were trying to reach the Waodani Indians deep in the jungles of Ecuador. One of the martyrs was his father, Nate Saint.

> "You know what my conclusion is? I don't think God merely tolerated my dad's death. I don't think He turned away when it was happening. I think He planned it. Otherwise I don't think it would have happened. This was a hard realization for me to come to. I once said that while speaking at a church, and a man came up afterwards and said, "Don't you ever say that again about my God.""

Afterward I found these verses in Acts 2:

> "Men of Israel, listen to these words. Jesus the Nazarene, a man attested to you by God with miracles and wonders and signs which God performed through him in your midst, just as

you yourselves know, you know he was God. You nailed him to a cross, you godless people. But he was delivered up to you by the predetermined plan of God." (vv. 22–23, AT)

Then I thought: Don't anybody tell me this can't be. If God could plan the death of His own righteous Son, why couldn't He plan the death of my dad?"[1]

When I contemplate the death of my little sister, Amie, laying it out again before God and asking for Him to continue to redeem it, I don't believe it was an accident. There is no way she died without God's knowing and planning it. She was legally blind. She found an unlocked door to the outside of the building and then she found a way to get off the fenced property. She was wandering about the golf course during daylight hours. She was apparently invisible, because no one saw her and intervened to keep her from drowning. I'm not sure you'll understand how it is comforting to me to know how many things had to fall perfectly into place for her to die; it couldn't have been random.

I am now much steadier in my trust of God, truly believing that "He is before all things, and in Him all things consist" (Colossians 1:17 NKJV). He is in control. I would rather know He is ultimately and intimately in control of everything than for even a brief second think He is somehow incapacitated by the ruler of this world. Satan cannot cause anything to happen that God has not ordained. And all that God does is for His glory. He knew all of us before we were formed in our mothers' wombs, and He knew the number of our days before even one of them began.

Ravi Zacharias penned these words:

"When God is our Holy Father, sovereignty, holiness, omniscience, and immutability do not terrify us; they leave us full of awe and gratitude. Sovereignty is only tyrannical if it is unbounded by goodness; holiness is only terrifying if it is un-tempered by grace; omniscience is only taunting if it is unaccompanied by mercy; and immutability is only torturous if there is no guarantee of goodwill. Thanks be to God, we know with a surety that His grace and goodness and hope and His love under-lie all of these attributes."[2]

Someday I'm going to better understand how the evil in the world is being worked together for the glory of God. In the meantime I know that Jesus cares about my pain. He fully empathizes with my heartache and the sense of injustice in this life. He promises it will all be made right. God not only promises to perfect me, but He also promises to perfect all things that concern me. The words of Psalm 138:8 fill me with this hope: "The LORD will accomplish what concerns me; Your lovingkindness, O LORD, is ever-lasting; do not forsake the works of Your hands" (NASB).

I do not have it all figured out, not by a long shot, but the redemption of my sister's life and death in the course of my life is unmistakable. Without all the suffering and tragedy I have endured, I would not have the empathy and compassion necessary to care for terminally ill children in my home. I have a hope of life beyond the grave—the hope of heaven and of life beyond this world. Make no mistake, if this life was it, I would not be doing what I do. But my God is good, my God is faithful, and He rewards those who seek Him and do what He commands. I mean it with my whole heart when I say I love these children who have been given to us for just a little time on earth, and I will indeed love them forever.

We invest deeply, and we ache terribly when these kids die, but our hearts are like stained glass windows made of broken glass that has been bonded back together. Those windows are even stronger and more beautiful for having been broken.

A FAMILY PERSPECTIVE

Here are some insights from a few more of my kids and Mark.

Charity, age 21

I've mentioned this often to my friends, and I'll say it again here: I think it's one of the coolest things that God makes babies cute. I mean, how much easier is it to take care of screaming children when they are super adorable? That is an aspect of God's work that I am very grateful for.

We started in this medical treatment foster care business with the cutest and easiest-to-love baby girl. So thank God for that one!

Although it was easy and fun to take care of Emmalynn, I remember being a little unsure of my mom's decision because Emmalynn was going to die and she needed a family to take care of her. Of course I was going to help! Because of the hope I have in Christ of eternal life in heaven, the idea of taking care of a baby who was going to die was much easier. I knew she was going to die, but I also believed she had heaven to look forward to. I wanted to love her even though I knew it would hurt when she died. I praise God for that kind of strength, because I know it wasn't my own.

Taking care of Emmalynn reminded me of what a family should be like. Or even more personally, what I should be like. My life should not be centered on only taking care of myself and no one else. God has called me to love Him and to love others. Taking care of Emmalynn reminded my family and me of how we are supposed to love others and not just ourselves.

Emmalynn's life and death were peaceful, and I do not regret in the slightest having taken care of her.

Fast-forward to taking care of Charlie. Charlie, though he has grown in his beauty, was not the cutest baby I had ever seen. Thankfully, looks do not mean that much to me when it comes to loving people. Charlie was a baby whom I knew we could care for because my siblings expressed willingness to do so and because my mom's nursing background gave us confidence that we could handle him. I'm so thankful we said yes as a family.

Charlie is one of the sweetest little kids I've ever been blessed to know. He doesn't communicate with his voice, but his eyes and his mannerisms speak volumes. I love watching movies with him; I love talking to him, holding his hand, kissing his adorable face, and including him in our daily activities. As you now know, Charlie was not expected to live to the age of two. This past spring I realized that he was going to be around for a while, and there was a sudden shift in my thinking. Instead of just living day to day, I started to make plans. Charlie's birthday is on June 25, and I decided to help him have new adventures. So, for his birthday, I bought him a swimming suit and we went out into the kiddie pool, filling it with a few inches of water. Our home is undergoing some construction, and the yard is mostly sand and dirt. How perfect! My sister Mary Elisabeth and I fashioned our own little beach in the backyard for Charlie to enjoy. My sister and I even joked about how Charlie needs to live long enough to be a ring bearer of our weddings someday. I still hold loosely to those plans, but as long as he's here with us, we're going to make the most of it!

A friend of mine recently showed me pictures of her nephew, who is also three. The pictures were adorable, but it also made my heart hurt a little bit when I remembered that Charlie is three and can't run around like this other little boy. Charlie doesn't complain, but I do wish he could be free from the constraints his body puts on him. However, just because he can't do those things doesn't mean he doesn't have ways to be a little kid. My family and I often joke about how we love Charlie's irritated face. Sometimes if he has been resting, we suddenly wake him up by saying his name or kissing his face. He will then wave his arms around to move us away. I tried to take a nap by him once, and the whole time he was moving his hand up and down my face. He knew he wasn't alone in his bed, and I don't think he wanted to share his space. Honestly, his irritated face is adorable and reminds us all of his great personality.

Before we took in any more foster care kids, my mom would bring it up to us as a family, and it was up to us to say yes or no. The song "All of Me" by Matt Hammit rang very true in my case. I could have chosen to be halfhearted. I could have said no and made it difficult for my family to take care of another child, but thankfully, God had me wholeheartedly agree each time.

Similar to my faith in Jesus Christ, I knew foster care had to be an all-or-nothing deal. Either I was going to give everything or I was going to look back on my life someday and regret how I didn't live or love fully.

Taking care of foster kids with my family has taught me some things:

1. Life isn't about yourself.
2. Babies, whether they are cute or scary looking, healthy or terminally ill, wanted or left to die, are valuable and need to be loved.
3. Big families can be embarrassing at times, but you should probably get over it now. No one is perfect. You're not perfect. Some will judge you, but others will be encouraging and gracious.
4. Have fun.
5. Work or hang out with people who have "different abilities." It's easier to be understanding and gracious to those who have disabilities if you spend more time with them.

Andrew, age 17

My brothers T-bear and Charlie are not just good-looking; they know how to impact the soul and make you think about your life!

Emily, age 15

One of nicest things about home is that when everyone is out of the house, I can play my music loud and clean up without anyone bugging me, and Charlie never seems to dislike it. One evening I was at home, the sun was starting to set, and everyone else was still at work or running errands. I cranked up our music machine, and Charlie was being adorable and wonderful as usual. I thought, *Man, this is great. Charlie will be fabulous while I clean up the place.* Funny enough, when I gave him a kiss on the cheek and went into the kitchen to clean, his pulse oximeter immediately started beeping. I left the kitchen to check on him, and as soon as I was near him, his sats were quiet and in perfect condition. I talked to Charlie about how I was going to clean the kitchen so he had to be a good boy. I gave him a kiss on the nose and went back to the kitchen again with my music still playing. About ten seconds later his pulse ox went off again. I waited for it to go back to normal, but it went off again and again, so I moved from the kitchen. But just like that, as soon as I reached him, his sats were normal.

I was slightly puzzled as to why the machine kept going off. I said to Charlie, "Buster Brown, I need to clean up the place a bit before everyone comes home, okay?" Charlie didn't respond with a yes, but he was fully awake, looking at me and swinging his hands. I thought he was good to go, and I made sure his sensor was working properly before I walked back into the kitchen. Twenty seconds later his pulse ox began to beep again and again and again. I was slightly annoyed, thinking I could have cleaned up the kitchen by now. I knew it was not coincidence that his pulse ox kept going off while I was away and was completely fine when I was by his side. I laughed, because I now believed that Charlie was setting it off on purpose. I had no idea how, but I acknowledged that he didn't want to be alone and would become annoyed when I left him, and that is why his heart rate would be so high. Therefore,

I stayed by Charlie yet tried to continue to be productive.

I got to wondering how long it had been since his diaper had been changed and thought I'd better check it. I was met with a soaked bottom. I thought, *Whatever*, and started to take off his diaper. I was not prepared, as I looked away to move some items that were in the way, for Charlie to make a huge poop that, ladies and gentlemen, got *everywhere*! On the floor, on his bed, on his toys—yep, *everywhere*.

Surprisingly, I wasn't annoyed, just grossed out. So as a way to trick my gag reflex into going away and to make the situation a bit lighter, I started speaking sarcastically in a British accent. I moved Charlie from his bed to his beanbag chair so I could clean up the mess. Everything that smelled went in the laundry room. In the meantime Charlie fell soundly asleep and my family returned home. I was torn between crying tears of joy upon seeing them and bursting out laughing at their reaction to the pile of soiled clothing, laundry, and toys and Charlie's wet mattress.

Johanna, age 23

Music is one of God's greatest gifts to His children, a gift that I love. It moves us, changes us, makes us feel more intensely than we would without it. Music can also be linked to memories, so every time you hear a certain song, you are brought back to that moment in your life and your emotions at that time. When God blessed my family with Emmalynn, music was a way to make memories with her that would still be with me after she died. Songs like "You Wouldn't Cry" by Mandisa and "I Will Carry You" by Selah reminded me that this world is not our home. That Emmalynn is a gift from God, and we are to love and cherish her while she is with us, miss her when she flies to heaven, and be excited for the day we will see her again. These songs now bring a peace to my heart that Emmalynn is more than fine. She is whole, beautiful, and loved, dancing and laughing before the Lord.

When Emmalynn came into my life, she changed me and changed our whole family. When God healed my mom, my family was made stronger. When He brought Emmalynn into our lives, it was made even more beautiful.

When I first met Charlie, I was scared and way outside my comfort zone, for I had decided years before that I was not cut out for a medical profession. I nearly fainted at a body museum. I don't like watching medical dramas or looking at or reading about medical procedures. Even medical lingo makes me uncomfortable. Since my mother and sister are both nurses, I couldn't avoid the topic completely, for they didn't seem to find anything wrong or uncomfortable about explaining in great detail things I think should be kept hidden. We have skin for a reason!

Nevertheless, I found myself agreeing to go with my mom to visit our Charlie for the first time. I was scared and knew it was going to be a challenge, but I was committed to step up and go through the training needed to bring him home. Charlie needed my family, and I knew God would give us the strength required for the task He called us to.

When I first saw Charlie, I was afraid to touch him for fear I would hurt him somehow. It didn't take long, though, for me to see the sweet little baby boy under all those wires and beeping machines. I fell completely in love with him. Even then it took weeks of holding him and months of training before I felt completely comfortable with him.

My mom and I spent so much time at Children's Hospital that the beautiful Ronald McDonald House really started feeling like our second home. The stunning Christmas decorations that year are a beautiful memory. Still thanking God for the incredible blessing that is Ronald McDonald House. I loved all the time with my mom and Charlie as we trained to bring him home.

It was a big challenge and tested our faith and pushed us all out of our comfort zones as we learned how to best care for Charlie. It was hard. Sometimes so hard that I didn't think we could do it. But God gave us strength to get through.

My mom is my hero and my inspiration. Even with the fear she must have felt being responsible for this child, her faith was apparent. The fear we felt to be responsible for Charlie was a daily reminder and invitation to lean into the One who is our strength and refuge. God called us to this; there is no question about that. He always gives us the strength for what He has called us to do.

My kids here at the orphanage in Thailand love Charlie, too, even though they've never met him.

Mark, old enough

Some people say that life is a journey or an adventure. I believe that. And there is a time and purpose for every season; and every experience and every person we interact with makes us who we are. So it certainly has been an adventure with Cori and our family. God has been good to us; yes, so very good.

To men reading this, I want to say to you specifically, "Never give up—*never*!" To win the prize, to have abundant life, to have the very best that God has planned for you, and to really live freely, *never* give up. Stay true to that promise you made to your wife before God, your family, and friends on your wedding day.

As Cori's health was at the darkest point and as she was lying on our bed in pain and in the fetal position, slowly dying, I was trying to maintain the home, go to work, homeschool the kids, and keep a hopeful and positive attitude with our children. It seemed like all the world was pressing down on our lives. I wept before God on many nights in what seemed a hopeless situation. Taking the high road with our children, I would often say to them, "Don't look at the dirt on the windows, but look past it and see the beauty of the day," while I myself was grieving inside.

What seemed to be the darkest night of the soul later proved to be the preparation for our hearts to do what we are doing now with suffering, seemingly hopeless, and sometimes abandoned children. I specifically remember one night in bed when Cori was maxed out on pain meds and she asked me, "Why do you stay with me?" My response was, "Because I love you, and one day you will know what that really means." That day has come.

Cori did miraculously recover, and that diamond in the rough has become a brilliant shining jewel for the love of God. And what potentially could have destroyed our family made us stronger, more compassionate, loving, and kind. I believe in miracles. God is good, and I have no regrets.

Our introduction into the foster care world was a little baby, a beautiful little angel, who got us out of hardened survival mode and taught us to love again. She lived fifty days and gave us more life than we ever could have given her. I am looking forward to the day in heaven when this beautiful little girl comes up behind me and says, "Daddy, it has been worth it all." You see, there is no turning back now. God loves these little living souls through us, and though loving them involves some tears, we also experience a sense of hope, life, and well-being that cannot be expressed in words. I feel God now more than ever in my life. I value the simple things that last forever. Truly there is an abundant life, and it doesn't consist in stuff.

Life is an adventure, so choose the road you are on and never quit.

NOTES

Chapter 2: Amie

1. David Powlison, quoted in John Piper and Justin Taylor, eds., *Suffering and the Sovereignty of God* (Wheaton, IL: Crossway, 2006), 156.
2. Kate Clifford Larson, *Rosemary: The Hidden Kennedy Daughter* (New York: Houghton Mifflin Harcourt, 2015), 176.

Chapter 3: Fifty Days

1. Ruth Hulburt Hamilton, "Song for a Fifth Child," *Ladies Home Journal,* October 1958, 186.
2. C. S. Lewis, *A Grief Observed* (New York: HarperCollins, 1994), 6.

Chapter 4: The Funeral

1. Angus Buchan, *Faith Like Potatoes* (Oxford: Monarch Books, 2006), 62–63.
2. Ibid.

Chapter 5: Flaws Revealed and Healed

1. *Masterpiece Classic: Downton Abbey*, season 1, episode 2, Brian Percival, Ben Bolt, Brian Kelly, Andy Goddard, James Strong, and Ashley Pearce (2010; Hampshire, England: Carnival Films and Masterpiece, 2010), DVD.
2. Timothy Keller and Kathy Louise Keller, *The Meaning of Marriage* (New York: Riverhead, 2011), 101.
3. Mental Health Act (Wisconsin 2005), accessed August 27, 2017, https://docs.legis.wisconsin.gov/2005/statutes/statutes/51.pdf, 11.
4. David Powlison, quoted in John Piper and Justin Taylor, eds., *Suffering and the Sovereignty of God* (Wheaton, IL: Crossway, 2006), 156–57.

Chapter 6: The Broken Vessel

1. John Piper, "How Do You Keep Going?" DesiringGod .org, June 17, 2001, www.desiringgod.org/messages /how-do-you-keep-on-going-for-130-years.

2. Jon Bloom, "Lay Aside the Weight of Perfection," DesiringGod.org, June 9, 2017, http://www.desiringgod .org/articles/lay-aside-the-weight-of-perfection.

Chapter 7: The Dark before the Dawn

1. Joni Eareckson Tada, quoted in John Piper and Justin Taylor, eds., *Suffering and the Sovereignty of God* (Wheaton, IL: Crossway, 2006), 196.

Chapter 8: The Tight Fist of Fear

1. Daniel Parker, *Phrenology and Other Poems* (Lowell, MA: S. W. Huse, 1859), 7.

2. Beth Moore, *Esther: It's Tough Being a Woman* (Nashville: LifeWay, 2008).

Chapter 10: Strength Made Perfect in Weakness

1. Pam Rosewell Moore, *Life Lessons from The Hiding Place: Discovering the Heart of Corrie ten Boom* (Grand Rapids: Chosen, 2004), 53.

2. Widely attributed to Corrie ten Boom. Original source unknown.

3. Wisconsin State Legislature, Statute 448.30, accessed August 3, 2017, https://docs.legis.wisconsin.gov /statutes/statutes/448/III/50.

Chapter 11: Crazy Amazing Answers to Prayer

1. Ravi Zacharias, *Cries of the Heart* (Nashville: Thomas Nelson, 2001), 25.

2. Anthony Hopkins, in character as C. S. Lewis, says this line in *Shadowlands*, a movie based on the play by William Nicholson. Taken from a transcript of the film's script. "Shadowlands," Script-o-Rama.com, accessed August 4, 2017, www.script-o-rama.com /movie_scripts/s/shadowlands-script-transcript-winger -hopkins.html.
3. Martha Snell Nicholson, "Treasures," in *Ivory Palaces* (Chicago: Moody, 1946).
4. Kate Clifford Larson, *Rosemary: The Hidden Kennedy Daughter* (New York: Houghton Mifflin Harcourt, 2015), 225.
5. Veryabc.cn, "Nobody's as handsome as David. . .not even David," *Sabrina*, directed by Sydney Pollack (Hollywood, CA: Paramount Pictures, 1995), accessed August 2, 2017.

Chapter 12: Stained Glass Windows
1. Steve Saint, quoted in John Piper and Justin Taylor, eds., *Suffering and the Sovereignty of God* (Wheaton, IL: Crossway, 2006), 117.
2. Ravi Zacharias, *Cries of the Heart* (Nashville: Thomas Nelson, 2001), 24.

Cori Salchert is a mother of fifteen kiddos and counting. She knows what it's like to love deeply, while holding loosely to the terminally ill children she cherishes in her home for the brief time they live before dying. Her strength and hope is in God, and the pain and grief endured on earth is worth it because she'll have forever to love her children in heaven.

Marianne Hering has been a writer and book editor in the Christian book market for more than 20 years. Her fiction series for children, The Imagination Station, has sold upwards of 500,000 copies. Currently, she works as the Senior Associate Editor of *Focus on the Family* magazine. Among the bestselling authors she's worked with are Dr. Greg and Erin Smalley, apologist Dr. Alex McFarland, and pastor Dr. Tony Evans. She lives in Colorado Springs with her husband and twin sons.

CONTINUE YOUR SPIRITUAL INSPIRATION WITH. . .

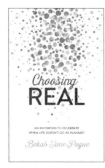

Choosing Real
by Bekah Jane Pogue

In *Choosing REAL*, author Bekah Pogue walks with women into life's unplanned circumstances—specifically frantic schedules, pain and transition, feelings of unworthiness, loneliness, and tension. . . And she reminds them it is in these very moments that God invites us to notice, respond, and even *celebrate* how He shows up—in every little detail.
Paperback / 978-1-63409-964-6 / $14.99

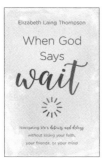

When God Says "Wait"
by Elizabeth Laing Thompson

Author Elizabeth Laing Thompson invites readers to walk alongside people of the Bible who had to wait on God. . .like David, Joseph, Miriam, and Naomi. Their stories will equip us to live our own stories—particularly our problematic waiting times—with faith, patience, perspective, and a healthy dose of humor.
Paperback / 978-1-68322-012-1 / $14.99

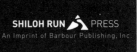